UNDERSTANDING
THE MESSAGES OF
YOUR BODY

Also by Jean-Pierre Barral

Visceral Manipulation (with Pierre Mercier)

Visceral Manipulation II

Trauma: An Osteopathic Approach (with Alain Croibier)

Urogenital Manipulation

The Thorax

Manual Thermal Evaluation

Manual Therapy for the Peripheral Nerves (with Alain Croibier)

Manual Therapy for the Cranial Nerves (with Alain Croibier)

UNDERSTANDING THE MESSAGES OF YOUR BODY

How to Interpret
Physical and Emotional Signals
to Achieve Optimal Health

North Atlantic Books
Berkeley, California

Upledger Enterprises
Palm Beach Gardens, Florida

Published by	and
North Atlantic Books	Upledger Enterprises
P.O. Box 12327	4521 PGA Boulevard, #245
Berkeley	Palm Beach Gardens
California 94712	Florida 33410

Cover and book design by Susan Quasha
Cover photo © istockphoto.com/angelo gilardelli
Printed in the United States of America

Understanding the Messages of Your Body: How to Interpret Physical and Emotional Signals to Achieve Better Health is sponsored by the Society for the Study of Native Arts and Sciences, a nonprofit educational corporation whose goals are to develop an educational and cross-cultural perspective linking various scientific, social, and artistic fields; to nurture a holistic view of arts, sciences, humanities, and healing; and to publish and distribute literature on the relationship of mind, body, and nature.

North Atlantic Books' publications are available through most bookstores. For further information, visit our website at www.northatlanticbooks.com or call 800-733-3000.

PLEASE NOTE: The creators and publishers of this book disclaim any liabilities for loss in connection with following any of the practices, exercises, and advice contained herein. To reduce the chance of injury or any other harm, the reader should consult a professional before undertaking this or any other martial arts, movement, meditative arts, health, or exercise program. The instructions and advice printed in this book are not in any way intended as a substitute for medical, mental, or emotional counseling with a licensed physician or health-care provider.

Library of Congress Cataloging-in-Publication Data

Barral, J. P.
  [Comprendre les messagers de votre corps. English]
  Understanding the messages of your body : how to interpret physical and emotional signals to achieve optimal health / by Jean-Pierre Barral.
      p. cm.
  Summary: "Describes the relationship between the emotions and the internal organs, with detailed analyses of various types of human personality and their related physical-emotional complexes and organ dysfunctions. Provides exercise recommendations, psychological approaches, and dietary plans for self-healing"—Provided by publisher.
  ISBN-13: 978-1-55643-679-6
  ISBN-10: 1-55643-679-3
  1. Medicine, Psychosomatic—Popular works. I. Title.
RC49.B375 2007
616.08—dc22
                                                            2007021849

5 6 7 8 9 10 11 VERSA 16 15 14 13 12

Acknowledgments

My best and warmest thanks to all those who, through their presence and support, helped me progress on the road to recognizing our body's messages:

Jean Arlot, Professor Georges Arnaud, Michel Boujenah, Marc Bozetto, Paul Chauffour, Professor Pierre Cornillot, Vincent Coquard, Françoise Coulet, Jacaues Descotte, Thomas Dummer, Didier Feltesse, Viola Fryman, Régis Godefroy, Barbara Hendricks, Lionelle Issartel, Bernard Lignier, Frank Lowen, Jean-Paul Mathieu, Pierre Mercier, Serge Paoletti, Professor Bernard Paramelle, Henri Pinel, Didier Prat, Louis Rommeveaux, Maurice-Paul Sainte-Rose, Dominique Thévenot, Dominique Triana, John Upledger, John-Matthew Upledger, Gail Wetzler, John Whernam, not to mention the Planchard and Igounet families and the entire Barral tribe, masterfully guided by Rose and René.

An additional thank you to Annabel Mackenzie and Dawn Langnes for their technical assistance in bringing the English version of this book to you.

CONTENTS

Introduction ᴧᴐ

Human beings are made up of a body and a mind. Every one of us is an individual, a unique entity. Before we come into the world, two beings must merge: we are the fruit of their union. Then we establish our own connection with our family and, later on, with society. We are part of the world, the universe, the cosmos … which are all in constant movement. We too are in perpetual motion. Everything in us, from birth until death, moves and changes. The processes of growth and aging are the clearest illustrations of this fact. To become aware of our own evolution, of the rhythms we are subjected to, of the movements that imprint themselves in us, of the different interconnections that make up a living body, is to learn to know and take care of ourselves so we can go through life in greater harmony.

Listening to Our Inner Self

This isn't to say that one should become a narcissistic egocentric! But you should never forget that you are the most important person in your life. Your own inner balance determines the balance of your environment, family, and social network. What you get in return will always be pure benefit. Therefore, it is your duty to yourself to monitor and maintain your health. Many people take better care of their car than they do their body. How many of those who enjoy humming along behind the wheel of a shiny car feel just as comfortable in their own skin? How many of those who run to the mechanic at the slightest suspicious noise in the motor go to the same trouble when they feel uncomfortable or unwell?

Let's not overdo listening to ourselves to the point of becoming hypochondriacs. But let us learn how to listen to our body and to its reactions, so we can be in tune with our "motor," to avoid breakdowns and to make the most of its capacities.

We all have our individual fears, our complex neuroses, our guilt feelings. Let's just take one step outside the limits we've locked ourselves into voluntarily and take a good look at ourselves, way down to the nitty-gritty. Let's look at what we all have in common, at the same time make the most of our differences, which enable each one of us to be a unique human being. We can transform our negative perceptions into constructive action.

Understanding Ourselves Better

Let's learn to stop being afraid of our body and its reactions. Let's allow ourselves to express our emotions. We mustn't forget that emotions affect our physical body. Understanding this is the first step toward a better life. We need to understand how our body stores trauma in its memory so that we can detect any forewarnings of dysfunction. Let us seek to prevent, rather than wait until we have to cure. Everyone feels better when they pay attention to their health. Parents go out of their way to instill practical and moral sense in their children, to teach them to get by in daily life, to integrate socially, to become "independent." Why not seek greater autonomy in managing our own health too? I think we should embrace positively the old saying "God helps those who help themselves," and learn to count primarily on ourselves in building up personal health. Know yourself, eat healthily, exercise—these are the basic precepts we need to follow to offer ourselves the joy of a well-functioning body and mind.

Achieving Better Health

The current premise of the health system in the West is "Be sick, we'll cure you." This may not be the best attitude. It would be better to advise, "First of all, do everything you can to stay healthy." Throughout this book, I'll do my best to give you information that will help you understand the language of your body and adapt to its requirements, so that you'll be in better shape and health. For instance, if you wake up one morning with pains in your stomach, before you run to the drugstore and buy pills to obscure the pain, ask yourself a few basic questions: What was my day like yesterday? Did I get into any clash with my superiors at work? If so, how irritated did I really feel? If you come to the conclusion, for example, that bitter words from your boss might have set off those stomach pains, you may not only reduce the pain, but also build up better defense mechanisms. How? By finding a new way of dealing with offensive occurrences, by strengthening your self-protection, by focusing on your strong points. By taking care of your organs through healthy food and lifestyle. A little bit of introspection can go a long way. Following an appropriate diet, avoiding toxins, practicing carefully chosen physical exercise, gentle techniques such as relaxation or yoga if necessary—all these contribute to building up a stronger defense system, which in turn will assist you in dealing with adversity, and creating a balanced state of health.

In order to achieve optimal health, one must focus on the role of the organs. In this book, for every organ you will find:

- A brief description of how it works.
- A more detailed explanation of its most common types of dysfunction and of possible symptoms.
- The emotions which are linked to it.
- A description of the personality and the emotional range that fit the organ. For example, you can be a "liver" or a "heart" or a "kidney" person. This is only a general tendency of course, since all our organs interact.
- Last but not least, how to care for the organ from a physical, nutritional, and psychological point of view.

Before running to a specialist who will say, "It doesn't look good, let's take care of you," don't forget that there are efficient measures you can practice yourself to preserve your own health: listening to and understanding the messages of your body.

PART ONE

Your Body Talks, Listen to It!

1

The Human Body,
A Well-Oiled Machine

The inside of our body is invisible to us. Beyond a few notions of anatomy and medicine, we do not know much about how the body functions and how its different systems interact. The great mystery of "our insides" is contained within an envelope—our skin—which works as a defense against outer aggressions, like the walls of a city. Our skin protects our life. Any breach of these ramparts puts us in danger. Any physical trauma, act of surgery, wound, or fracture is a destructive action that weakens us. Wounds heal, but the skin will bear a visible scar, and the inside of the body retains the invisible memory of scars, pain, and stress. These underlying tensions can resurface at any moment.

Psychological aggression and trauma create a more insidious breach of our defenses, going through them without leaving any apparent traces. No superficial scar tissue results—but a memory imprints itself deep down inside the body. Its first target will be our "weak link," our most sensitive spot or vulnerable organ. It can be the back, the liver, the intestine…. Furthermore, our bodies give off electromagnetic fields that build another guard (or shield) around our skin, a subtle and invisible one. You'll be aware of it when someone comes too close. It is that feeling of "this is as close as I want to be to that person," the feeling of the distance we need to keep between ourselves and the other person to keep him or her from "invading our space."

This breach, whether visible or invisible, becomes like a leak in a boat. The crew does its best to seal it off: with a healthy crew, the damage will be repaired in no time. But if the crew is exhausted from having just been through several days of rough sea or dealing with mechanical problems, it may be beyond their capacity to fix the problem. The leak could end up sinking the ship simply because the crew lacked the energy!

In Our Organs, the Echo of our Emotions

When we feel an emotion, it is not our foot or our chin reacting, but our organs. They are extremely receptive to our emotions and feelings. This is how our emotions "take shape." We express this spontaneously in everyday language: "Stop your bellyaching," "It makes me want to throw up," "I have a gut feeling," "This gives me heartburn," "That left me breathless" or "… gave me goose-bumps," etc. You'll also hear "He has guts," "She wears her heart on her sleeve," and similar expressions.

We have a rich vocabulary to describe the emotional range of our organs. There is a certain hierarchy in the way our organs react. It depends on the intensity, the severity, and the duration of the stress they encounter. You can't compare the stress caused by the loss of a set of keys to the loss of a job or a breakup with a loved one.

The usual classification, in order of degree, puts the death of a loved one in first place, then divorce, the loss of a job, an undesired move, followed by an endless list. Emotional reactions range from simple spasms in the gallbladder to heartburn, vomiting, feeling faint, actually fainting, ulcers, hepatitis, and more serious diseases. Usually, with small annoyances, it is the gallbladder and the solar plexus (located at the center of the stomach) which react. All our organs are physically and emotionally connected to the brain. The emotional relationship with the brain is a qualitative one since the brain isn't affected physically to the same extent as other organs are by various types of stress. The intestine and the liver, the greatest "hoarders" of emotion, definitely get first prize.

In Our Behavior, the Echo of Our Organs

Not only do organs react to emotions, but an organ's reaction can determine a behavioral pattern. Take the intestine, for example, which is often related to psychological rigidity and a cleanliness phobia. When a person with a fragile or weak intestinal system is going through a crisis, he or she may suddenly go on a cleaning binge or get angry at people over nothing.

Our Weak Link

We are not equal where visceral dysfunction is concerned. Every person has his or her weak link, an organ or body part that is more vulnerable than the others and becomes the main target of stress. Sometimes people are aware of their weak link or "Achilles heel." There is often a genetic predisposition to weakness of a particular organ. Or it may have become weak due to an unhealthy lifestyle. For example, someone with a sensitive liver will have a hard time the morning after a rich meal or too much alcohol. He'll be grumpy, irascible, aggressive; the slightest bit of stress will irritate him. Whoever crosses his path that day should watch out! A futile pretext might spark off an overheated argument.

To add to the complexity of the human body's workings, it should be said that in the wide world of emotions, every organ has its favorite terrain. We'll analyze them specifically further on, but here are a few simple examples to illustrate:

- The liver is sensitive to everything pertaining to the unity of our being, to our deepest self.
- The spleen and the pancreas are particularly vulnerable during intense, intolerable emotional states, caused by external events such as the accidental death of a loved one.
- In women, the breasts react to family problems, and to a lack of stability and affection. They can become congested, painful, or develop cysts or tumors.
- With men, the stomach often reflects social life. It collects the tensions that arise in the course of conflict with other people.
- When affected by stress, certain organs such as the bronchial passages, the stomach, the gallbladder, or the intestines can be subject to spasms.
- With other organs, such as the kidneys, it is mainly the vascular and excretory systems which tense up, leading to dysfunction of the organ itself.

- Like a shock wave, stress resonates in different parts of the body. But the human being can resort to a range of preventive measures to ensure that his or her "inner being" stays in good shape and functioning well.

The human body is not just a machine. It is constantly recording stimuli and input and experience. We carry within us the memory of our ancestors. This is our genetic heritage. It can be strength or longevity we inherit, but it can also be more or less apparent illnesses, such as allergies, diabetes, asthma, psoriasis, or eczema—hidden illnesses which lurk, waiting to be reborn, like lava beneath a volcano. An emotionally stressful situation can reawaken an unsuspected genetic disease.

A twenty-five-year-old patient came to me with terrible eczema that had appeared suddenly two days before. I knew that she was very sensitive. Did she go through some kind of emotional shock? With a long sigh, as if the sky were falling on her head, she said, "No, no shock, but I had a job interview last week. I was incredibly stressed out." I asked her if anyone in her family is prone to eczema. "My grandmother," she replied. She carried the seed in her. It developed under the pressure of the job interview, her first big stress situation as a responsible, adult woman.

The Brain

The brain is the inseparable link between the body and the spirit. It receives, transmits, and memorizes. It allows us to think, to imagine, to create, to talk and to walk. It is the brain that decides whether we should be happy or unhappy, whether we should laugh or cry, be active or inactive. This 2.87 pounds of cerebral matter is a long way from having revealed all its secrets! Thinking, transmitting, and producing, the brain is the relay between our connection to the cosmos and the concrete reality of our body. The biological and seasonal rhythms (circadian, or the sun's rhythm, and monthly or moon rhythms) transit through the brain before they begin to influence the way the body functions.

Given that it is only two percent of the body's total weight, the brain is a great oxygen consumer, utilizing twenty percent of the body's oxygen (ten times more than other parts of the body). The best way to bring oxygen to the brain is to be physically active. Once you know that the brain commands muscles, extremities, nerves, hormones, reactivity, thought, and will, you realize that the body is a highly developed mechanism that regulates itself but is not autonomous. To function properly, the body needs input from the outer world and various types of stimuli. The essence is nutrition, then comes psychological input. Affection, recognition, self-esteem, and intellectual work are some of the factors that promote balance.

62,000 Miles of Nerves

The brain and the entire body are in constant communication. The slightest bit of information sets off a whole communications system composed of nerves which function like a network of miniature cables. These cables travel across our entire body and connect in two central areas: the spinal cord and the brain. If we were to arrange all our nerves in one line, they would be 62,000 miles long. That is about two and a half times around the Earth. This number in itself illustrates the complexity of the human body. Furthermore, every nerve has a corresponding artery. So our body is also laced with 62,000 miles of arteries. Such a perfect system, whose origins escape our knowledge, should encourage us to remain modest in regard to the exceptional gift that nature has given us.

Thank Goodness, We Have Psychosomatic Reactions!

The brain is in charge of psychosomatic reactions that are actually a rather healthy way of getting rid of our psychological burdens. The brain receives so much information that it cannot store it all without paying a price. Normally, if you include all five senses, the brain receives up to ten billion pieces of information per second. When in danger, a hundred million extra stimuli instantaneously assail it. Fortunately, all this information gets sorted out and put in order by a nervous structure called the reticulate "substance" or "formation." Psychosomatic phenomena occur when emotional residue pours into our organs. As long as this process remains within acceptable boundaries and doesn't put our lives in danger, it is a positive phenomenon that helps us maintain our mental health. Outside acceptable boundaries we experience pain and discomfort.

Rather like the chicken and egg question of which came first, one must try to discover what is promoting the pain. Sometimes it appears that pain originates with an emotional upset, which then creates distress in an organ. Sometimes an organ is physically damaged, and this is what in turn stimulates emotional traits (associated with that organ) to emerge.

Because joints, muscles, and ligaments share certain nerve centers with particular organs, irritation in an organ can cause a problem in a joint. The inverse also applies: a problem in a joint can set off a problem in an associated organ. Treating either component will help to bring about greater health in the person. Treating both aspects will ensure optimal well being.

Sometimes—because we are preoccupied and we think too much, because we imagine and we dramatize—we blow up small events. For example, a patient came to see me for recurring and increasingly troublesome back pain. Nothing abnormal appeared in scans and MRI. But instead of being reassured by this fact, she imagined the worst. She had become depressed over her back problems and was suffering from digestive trouble. We've all heard that little insidious voice whispering to us: "You may be in danger; cancer can start that way." The recurring pain awakens the anguish of disease and death, which are inherent to humankind. In the course of the session, working with her thorax and ribs revealed that a rib on her left side, quite far from the spine, was completely fixated; it did not move. When I pressed this particular point, the pain was evident: "That is exactly where it hurts!" she exclaimed. "How did you find it?"

It is not by questioning the person that we find the problem, but by asking the body and interpreting its messages. Painful areas literally draw the therapist's hand toward them. The doctors that this patient had seen focused on her spinal cord. In fact, the rib fixation occurred through a movement she made when closing her shutters. This physical problem led to dysfunction of the pancreas, which in turn contributed to her state of anxiety. This case illustrates the importance that a small event in daily life can assume in a weakened person. We all over-dramatize a little sometimes, and even more if the therapist doesn't understand us, or isn't able to feel or analyze our pain. Not to have one's pain recognized causes anguish and frustration.

2

Emotions for Life

Emotion expresses itself. It can be read on a person's face: eyes shine for joy, the mouth opens in astonishment. Emotion can be visible on the skin: we blush, turn pale, get goose-bumps. Our gestures as well can indicate emotion: we raise our hands to our face in fear. Even before speech appeared, emotional communication was the primitive person's first way of exchanging and communicating. Originally it came from within, just like animal instinct. With civilization and the sophistication of our habits, human beings learned to control their emotions. But we still jump for joy, laugh in happiness, smile with pleasure, cry in sorrow, and show vexation on our face, to name only a few ways that emotion is displayed. According to our education and environment, we may more or less repress and internalize our emotions. Yet a person who could hide his or her entire emotional range would be quite an oddity. It would be a grave error for his or her psychological balance, at any rate. We are not all equal before emotion, and we have not all been to the same school when it comes to reacting to events.

The Great Spectacle of Our Emotions

Remember the young British soccer fan who lived up to his challenge to streak naked across the field during a widely publicized major-league game? From our TV viewer's seat, it was interesting to watch the public's reactions. Some people shouted, laughed, gestured, and clapped, while others stood up, their mouths agape in astonishment; others remained seated, their faces stony with disapproval. Some people even seemed frightened, covering their mouth with one hand while pointing with the other at the

9

police squad approaching the guy. The same stimulus can touch off very different reactions in different individuals. What fills some people with joy can make others anxious. Every person reacts with his or her own emotional tenor, cultural traditions or "biases," and education.

Emotion: Between Reason and Impulse

We can more or less control many of the physical mechanisms linked to our emotions. For example, breathing deeply relaxes the muscles and slows down the heart rate. It is by making an effort to understand our impulses that we can manage them better, regulate them, and achieve dominion of thought over emotion. This attitude only becomes natural to us after a long training process! We cannot totally eliminate emotion, but it is good to avoid excesses. The solution is within. There are several methods that can help us with this (see page 43). We will all attain different results because, as we know, we are not all equal in the face of emotion.

For a long time, IQ (intelligence quotient) was considered to be the only standard measure of intelligence. EQ (emotional quotient) is now acknowledged to be a factor. Two individuals with identical IQ and supposedly capable of understanding and solving the same problem will not make the same decision because their emotional reactivity is different. Why is this so? Simply because we are not robots, and every person has his or her own complex set of emotional reactions. If we look at the most extreme cases, a person's emotional makeup can be either very impulsive or curbed by education. According to how active or contained it is, emotion can help individuals progress, can keep them at a standstill, or worse yet, make them regress.

Antonio Damasio, an American neurologist and researcher and an international expert on emotions, asserts that our intellectual and moral judgments are determined by our emotions, and that our feelings result from our becoming conscious of certain emotions. In short, Damasio says that emotions precede reason and that they are interdependent. When circumstances set off an intense emotional reaction, very few people can stay in control. That is when our deep emotional nature and innermost, inborn being reveal themselves.

Emotion: The Cement We're Built With

It is said that experience builds character. To be more specific, it is mainly the emotions we go through in the course of our experiences that contribute toward forming our personality. When our experiences have been painful, we speak of trials. Faced with a similar test, two individuals will react and evolve differently. At an unconscious level, our deep-seated emotions take over the game and determine its outcome, as the following example shows. Two brothers lost their mother, at ages twelve and fourteen. They were raised by their father, who remarried soon after losing his first wife. Twenty years later, the older son is married and becomes the father of a newborn baby. He has a positive attitude with regard to his child's future. The second son is single and sickly. He complains of various ills, lives with a strong sense of injustice, and bears a grudge against life. From birth, the two sons did not display the same psychological aptitude. "When they were little, they had very different characters," says their father. "Strangely, when their mother died, the more passive one reacted with a fighting spirit, whereas the one who had seemed stronger-willed collapsed."

How can behavior undergo such a radical change, even in such young individuals? It is believed that by seven years of age, our personality is largely determined and parental education more or less complete. In our pre-teen years, we add educational and moral values to our genetic makeup: this is the fine-tuning of our emotional character, which was already unique from the start.

Everything the individual comes equipped with and everything that he or she acquires in the course of life is recorded in the body, like on a DVD or videotape, in picture and sound. For example, in the case of an accident, you have shock, with its plethora of pain and emotions. Time goes by, we think we've forgotten, but if we happen to be exposed to a similar stress situation again, present and past reconnect and can reawaken the old fear, because the movie of the past event is stored in our memory. One of my patients had a bike accident. A dog ran in front of her wheels and she hit the brakes too suddenly, locking the wheels and throwing her over the handlebars onto the road. At the same moment, she heard the sound of a truck coming up behind her. Not knowing where she had landed, she was terrified of being run over. But the truck wasn't actually that close to her. She suffered a fractured jaw and cervical sprain. At a much later time I treated her for recurring headaches. She had never imagined that these headaches could be linked not only to mechanical factors, but to the memory of the accident stored in her cervical vertebrae. But she told me that whenever she would hear a truck coming up behind her when riding her bike, she would be so paralyzed with fear that she would prefer to let herself fall into a ditch. Fear had left a stronger mark than pain.

A Four-Tiered Pyramid

An individual is based on a four-level structure:
- the inner self: what we are born with and what we are to become;
- the family, which develops our affect, shapes our character, instills precepts and values;
- society, into which the individual has to integrate, thereby receiving new initiations and facing difficulties;
- the individual himself or herself, a growing symbiosis of the inborn and the acquired.

The Body Has Its Own Memory

Among other things, the body retains the memory of trauma, whether it be physical or emotional. Physical trauma is direct. It hurts and causes an immediate reaction in the body, through the pain it sets off. The brain records both the bodily pain and the emotion attached to it at the same time. Everything is stored in our psychological and physical unconscious mind:

- genetics: diabetes, allergies, psoriasis, asthma, auto-immune diseases;
- fetal life: deficiencies, infections, malformations, mechanical constraint *in utero;*

- vaccinations: they can sometimes cause allergic reactions in sensitive people;
- the numerous infections we have contracted in the course of our life;
- physical trauma: falls, fractures, sprains, surgical acts, accidents;
- psycho-emotional trauma: linked to the family, education, friends, partners (divorce, separation, muggings, etc.);
- social trauma: unemployment, insecurity, social and professional problems;
- pollution, poor diet, etc.

Trauma will leave its mark. Negative emotional shocks such as fear, tension, stress, frustration, anger, demands, and guilt all transit through the brain, which passes on the information wherever it can. Organs are an excellent receptacle. It's the "hot potato" story: it burns, and whoever has it passes it on as quickly as possible to his neighbor. This is what the brain does with its neighbors, the organs. Emotions that are either too strong or not strong enough impact our organs. Depending on how violent the trauma is, our defense system might fight back, feel destabilized, or actually fall apart. Thus, just like with physical imbalances, an emotional imbalance can lead to dis-ease in a related organ. Addressing the cause of emotional upset will assist in decreasing the noxious stimuli that is bombarding the organ. By the same token, treating the affected organ with Visceral Manipulation (a manual therapy technique) can often do much to soften the intensity of an emotional upheaval.

The unconscious mind can record an accident in two-thousandths of a second. When such an event occurs, there are visible wounds that we can feel and treat, but there is also the fear, whose itinerary from the brain to the organ remains a secret to us. It goes its way, imprinting in the unconscious mind the slightest little memories of the circumstances: smells, sounds, movements, agitation, immobility, the heavy, muffled silence. As a consequence of an accident, the body can produce a recurrent urinary tract or lung infection, for example. Over time, this infection can lead to a weakness of the organ involved, leaving it more susceptible to stress in the future.

The Hand Can Feel Physical and Emotional Tensions

Properly trained therapists can locate the weakened physical element in an ailing person through manual contact. They will let their hand glide over the patient's body with a pressure equal only to the weight of their hand. Their hand will unfailingly be attracted toward the problem zone. The mechanical attraction of tissues magnetizes the hand. To sense emotional stress zones, the hand has to apply very light touch, almost as if losing contact. Laid on the head, the hand will also be drawn like a magnet to the area where the brain stores its strongest emotional tensions. The bodyworker's profession is empirical. This is why we need many more objective scientific experiences to be sure that we are not going off on the wrong track.

Organs have their own memory of stored emotions, which can materialize as disease whenever a new stress situation comes up. "As long as he'll be mortal, man will never be totally relaxed," Woody Allen said, with his usual "angst"-full humor. It is true that we all hide repressed fears deep down inside. Human beings have largely forgotten the ancestral fears that kept us vigilant in the face of natural aggressions back in Neolithic times: fear of fire, of storms, of wild animals, of death. As human life grew in complexity and sophistication, we developed new, more insidious fears.

3

What Do Our Organs Think?

Can our organs think? Isn't this our brain's job? Don't worry, the brain is still in charge of our thought processes. But our organs and brain have close nervous and hormonal connections, and they work together. In intense stress situations, the brain passes the excess stress on to the organs, whose fibrous matter immediately records the emotion. This sets off a psychosomatic reaction. It can be a stomachache, a headache, vomiting, diarrhea, or constipation, etc. Stress and psychosomatic phenomena occur simultaneously. Our brain and our organs react as one entity. Actually, the human body is the seat of a permanent "emotion-organ-behavior-organ" cycle.

Does every emotion affect an organ? Consider this definition of "emotion" in a medical dictionary: "intense or painful psychological reaction that powerfully affects numerous organs." So the medical world is aware of the fact that emotions have an impact on organs.

Can an organ influence our behavior? A dysfunctional organ can block our entire metabolism and exhaust us. It affects our energy, our sensitivity, our susceptibility, even traits of our intrinsic character. Every individual has a general energy potential, along with one organ that is more reactive or sensitive than the others, that infamous weak link. When the slightest failing occurs, the body adapts, using all the tools at its disposal to re-establish a balance. If the failing recurs frequently in the same organ, the body gets weaker and weaker, and the person's attitude changes. Here is a simple example. You have dinner at a restaurant. The food doesn't agree with you, and a few hours later you have heartburn and stomach pains. The next morning when you wake up, you don't feel

15

well, your complexion is blotched, and your stomach upset. You don't feel rested, you feel tense. At work, one of your colleagues makes some remark about a job you are just about to finish. To your colleague's great surprise, you overreact, becoming angry and irrational. Suppose now that one of your organs is chronically overburdened or weakened. Your behavior will be noticeably affected.

Conversely, can behavior influence an organ? Let's imagine, for instance, that you are excessively needy of affection and recognition—a character trait that "goes straight to the heart." It is as if your heart were always on the lookout, waiting for signs of affection from everybody around you. This need is so pervasive that your heart reacts to the slightest emotion. You put constant demand upon it, both emotionally and physically. Because of the excess stimulus, the heart becomes oversensitive and can develop abnormalities in rhythm or cause arterial spasms in the coronary arteries. Yes, indeed, behavior influences organs. Of course, some people might retort that there has to be a genetic predisposition, a constitutional problem. But this doesn't change the behavior-organ equation we're talking about.

"Psychological suffering can cause very real physical pain, often mistaken for a heart attack. When in shock, the heart muscle experiences spasms, which cause painful contractions in the chest, obstruction of the lungs, and breathing difficulties as well as shooting pains in the arms." —*New England Journal of Medicine,* as quoted in *Impact Médecin*

Many know this as the "broken heart" syndrome, which is caused by emotional stress and linked to adrenaline and noradrenaline pouring into the blood. This can be fatal if the subject already suffers from heart disease. In healthy subjects, the symptoms disappear within a few days.

Body, Mind, Same Story!

It works both ways: by treating the mind, we can influence the body. If we treat the body, we influence the mind. The main thing is to be able to identify which of the two is the real cause of the dysfunction. The brain itself is an organ too, subject to its own physiological disorders. Today we know that certain psychological diseases are not only caused by psychological factors as we used to think, but they can be the result of chemical and hormonal imbalance.

When something goes wrong with one of our organs, we are surprised, although there often is a logical explanation. Dysfunction is the body's way of expressing the tensions we harbor. We can make an analogy with a car: One morning you turn the ignition key and the motor doesn't react. You get angry at your vehicle. But give it a thought: maybe you forgot to take the car for a check-up recently. Remember those funny little noises it's been making for some time now? All that neglect! The engine was due to fail at some point. It's the same thing with your body, which is (let's not forget) a precious and intricate machine. Take this example: Out of the blue, lumbago immobilizes your back. Are you sure you didn't get any warning signals? A slight muscular backache in the morning when you woke up? Oh, yes, and that cramp the other day too, when you picked up that heavy bag. True, you say to yourself, I should have paid more attention to that. Then you remember that you fell on your coccyx a few years ago. You didn't worry too much about it at the time, but you did have some intestinal trouble that night. And the next day you had a hard time getting up, because of the stiffness in your spine, which "remembered" the shock, of course (although you didn't realize that). You were taking risks for the future by not paying attention to those very first symptoms.

Potential Weaknesses

Nobody is totally intact. We've discussed the fact that everyone has a weak link, a fragile zone. We all have a pathological potential we inherited from our ancestors or developed through our own lifestyle. Onto our genetic memory we layer family habits (poor eating habits, for one) and personal habits (smoking, for example) which our body registers. Added to this are our memories of trauma and our emotions. All this put together, accumulated over a lifetime, can unbalance a human being's capacity to function. Illness, be it physical or psychological, evolves over time. While the disease takes its time to form, it can appear suddenly. We are more receptive to bacteria and viruses when we are tired, weak, or irritated. Why do only fifteen percent of a given population develop the flu during an epidemic? It is because those people have a weaker constitution: weakness of the lungs, enfeeblement due to age, psychological or nutritional factors, lack of exercise.... Slight fatigue, a sudden cold, feeling discouraged for a moment—all these are symptoms not to be neglected at the onset of winter. Of course, other less obvious factors can contribute to creating a pathological condition. But there is no doubt that a healthy lifestyle and a vigilant attitude toward the body are indispensable to preserving health.

Is Life an Extravagant Coincidence?

Let's imagine our conception. Wasn't our very chance of coming into being minute? In her reproductive life-span, a woman produces about four hundred thousand ova. At the instant of conception, the man emits around eighty million sperm, and the ovum, on that miraculous day, only retains one. An extraordinary meeting, that of an ovum and a sperm, both endowed with a unique genetic memory that is to become our personal foundation as an individual. To be conceived is an extraordinary event. This capital was given to us, and we should take care of it to the best of our ability.

Too Much or Not Enough

The body is endowed with a two-speed nervous system: the accelerating system and the slowing-down system (the sympathetic and the parasympathetic systems). The accelerator intensifies the organs' reactions, whereas the slowing-down system dampens them. That is why an organ can react to stress in a totally contradictory way. This principle—either "too much" or "not enough"—can be seen in different types of reaction.

Imagine that you are walking with a group of people in the forest, and a snake suddenly crosses your path. You won't all react in the same way to this particular danger. Some of you will be paralyzed with fear, while others will run away and leave the danger behind. A few rare individuals will face the danger and chase the snake away or kill it. A similar event can set off opposite emotional reactions in different individuals. We've all been through stage fright before an exam or performance. This type of stress often affects our intestines. But in some people it will cause diarrhea and in others, constipation. Stage-fright victims, you have a choice between overflow and retention!

A "too much" person or a "not enough" person will usually, by nature, react in the corresponding manner. But sometimes, faced with a particularly powerful or unknown stress situation, the individual tendency can suddenly reverse. That's the paradox of being human! It is important to remember that whenever there is stress, there will inevitably be a reaction to the stress, and this reaction has repercussions for our behavior and consequently on our organs.

Such extreme organ imbalances will necessarily bring similarly extreme behavioral disorders. The fear that initiates diarrhea or constipation can also, on a behavioral level, bring on logorrhea (excessive talkativeness) or total silence. There are those who talk and those who remain silent, the angry types and the reserved types. It is easy to see how the organs can react in such divergent manners: overflow or blockage, as described above.

Depression—At the Far End of "Too Much" or "Not Enough"

Depression is a perfect illustration of the "too much" or "not enough" theory—a depressed person reacts too intensely to the stress he or she is exposed to. Depression can also be induced by a family gene. It can be a chemical imbalance in the brain: the compensation reaction that would allow the subject's balance to be restored is blocked or impeded. Although for a long time it was thought that psychological factors alone were responsible for depression, we now believe that the chemistry in the brain can be the trigger: imbalance in the neurotransmitters, a lack of vitamins or too acid a pH, for example.

There are also mechanical factors that can underlie depression. When depression occurs following skull concussion, properly trained manual therapists can help by decompressing the joints in the skull. Do you know that the bones in the skull can move? We're talking about a very slight general mobility that can get constricted, for example, if we wear too tight a hat. This movement is made up of minute dilatation and retraction, about fifty microns. The skull performs about ten thousand movements a day. When deprived of its freedom of movement, the skull can be the cause of a general lack of vitality in the body. It has indeed been observed that depressed people have very little skull movement. Certain manual therapy techniques can get the skull moving again, restoring well-being to the entire organism.

Fifty microns isn't much, but an experienced hand can detect these movements. By skimming over a painted surface, one can feel a coat of paint only four microns thick. Our senses have exceptional capacities that can be revealed if we train them. Wine-tasters, perfume-smellers and musicians who have perfect pitch prove this point. It's the same thing with the sense of touch.

4

Your Body Speaks, Listen to It

The body speaks a language we are not really familiar with. Certainly our forebears in the past few centuries did not learn to listen to it. On the contrary, in many societies the body was hidden: if something was wrong, you weren't supposed to listen to your inner voice but instead to "heal pain with pain," and if things got worse, you put yourself in the hands of science, without asking any questions. Because our education kept us ignorant of our bodies for so long, we are estranged from the intimate comprehension of its language. When everything is fine, the body simply exudes health and balance, through physical vivacity and a beaming personality. But like the beauty of a rose, this harmony is fragile. As we have seen, from the very beginnings of life the body is subjected to various aggravations the most common of which are childhood diseases, birth trauma, and other physical distress due to the fetal position *in utero*. Then on to the teen years, with their acne, heartbreaks, and confusing changes of puberty—normal physical or psychological worries that we end up forgetting but which do leave their mark.

With more serious problems, the resonance is greater. The body shouts in pain or revolt. Without our knowing why, words become wounds. So let us listen to this body of ours. But watch out! Pay attention but don't obsess over it. Take care of yourself but do not become a hypochondriac!

Life Is Not Always a Long Quiet River

Some people manage to hide their anxieties or to compensate for their imbalances. But how long can we keep up false appearances? There always comes a time, an event, where masks fall and nature shows its real face. Nothing is all white or all black, nothing is fixed. We go through constant physical transformations, the mind and spirit evolve, our character changes, and our sensitive organs—our weak links—might shift throughout our lifetime. This is why it's important to build up our strength, and to do so we need to know ourselves very well. Jean de La Fontaine wrote, "To know oneself well is the first and foremost of our cares."

"Let us not neglect anything our body tells us" is a principle that should be part of our education, from the youngest years on. We should learn to live with our body and emotions without fear, without repression, and without negligence, giving our health capital its rightful value. Our body is our property, and it is our duty to take care of it. Just like the farmer who keeps a watchful eye on his fields in order to encourage them to flourish, we can be watchful to maintain a healthy body and a radiant frame of mind. Every patch of land has its little inadequacies. So do we. We are not here to judge; we are here to understand and to adapt.

Variable Degrees of Resistance

When a plane enters a zone of turbulence, the passengers get shaken up and often worry. We also go through trouble zones in our lives. They shake us up and leave a negative trace in our brain (our "black box"). If trials pile up with no hope in sight of things getting better, we're in danger. Inevitably, a succession of psychological hardships will weaken us. We end up breaking down. Adventurous athletes who take on big challenges all know this. Damaged equipment, avalanches, storms, the cold, frostbite, cuts, loneliness, fatigue, lack of sleep—all these discouraging factors, when they accumulate, can lead to a big "nervous breakdown."

In regular daily life, there's no need to be a hero to be acquainted with the infernal spiral of excess emotional burden. When everything is going wrong, at some point (there's no telling when because it depends on your degree of resistance), the slightest problem or annoyance can be enough to make you break down. Your day wore you out—you encountered different problems and annoyances, and not a friendly soul around to give you support. You go home, hoping to relax. You know you'll find comfort with your family. You're considering going off skiing over the weekend, and you're pleased with the idea of getting your equipment ready for tomorrow. Unfortunately, you can't find the key to the basement where you keep your skis and shoes. Seeing how tense you are, your wife and children try to help you find the key. You don't even notice their good will. Everyone is bustling around you, which makes you even more anxious (but of course inertia would have been just as bad). You get angry, and a clash ensues, with big-time drama for a silly little problem that would have ended up being solved anyway. But it was that "last straw" that finally cracked the resilience of your nervous system.

Understanding without Fear

This book aims to help ease your apprehensions about what may be happening in your body and familiarize you with the subtleties of how we tick. And as we saw above, it will help you understand the relationship between your emotions and your organs. Every organ is characterized by a whole gamut of emotions and attitudes. I'll draw a picture of a different person portraying each organ, whether it be the liver, intestines, gallbladder, etc. This will assist you in understanding each organ as an emotional "person."

By the same token, if an actual person has a certain organ as his/her weak link, in this book they will also be known as that type of organ person, e.g. liver person, heart person. This will explain common traits that a person with that weak link might commonly express. The extent of weakness in the organ will determine how many or to what degree the person will portray the noted traits.

If you are experiencing some of the emotions or concerns related to specific organs, this is an opportunity to examine your health—mental and physical. Most of us may be able to relate to more than one organ person, and in varying degrees. What is your body conveying to you? Are there changes that would be helpful to make in your physical, nutritional and psychological world that would bring you greater health?

Of course, no single person ever displays all the physical or psychological symptoms related to a specific organ. Every organ has its own emotional specificity, but it can't claim sole dominion over a category of emotions or behavior. The organ can react in the "too much" or "not enough" range. For instance, an emotion affecting the intestine can cause constipation or violent diarrhea. Having studied hundreds of cases of people suffering from problems in the same organ, I've detected certain tendencies which attract or spark off similar types of emotions. Analyzing an emotion is not an exact science. We're a long way from mathematical diagrams. It is impossible to cast a person in a rigid emotional type-frame. Sometimes our own emotions surprise us. This book can help you detect early warning symptoms of declining health which could become more serious if you don't pay attention to them. If an organ gives you a little signal, take extra care of it and, generally speaking, of yourself! Learn to look for the cause. Learn to distinguish between the physical and the psychological aspects of all the different connections in your body.

We all create dis-ease in our bodies. Depending on what organs are affected, we have different experiences. One time we may be more like a "liver person," and another time we may react more like a "stomach person." In addition, we all have varying areas and degrees of genetic weakness. This is one reason why the same stressor can affect two people in very different ways. Certainly when stressed we typically experience greater discomfort in these weak links. Often the areas of genetic weakness will be more influenced when we have a systemic strain than in the event of stress arbitrarily impacting a specific part of the body. In the case of our genetic organ weak links, we would do well to understand these organs and what we can do to maintain their optimal health.

Healing an Emotional Problem by Treating an Organ

Take the case of someone who loses his or her job and suffers from stomach pains. This is what happens. The brain receives a negative message. It gets rid of it by sending it on to the stomach. This somatization (the expression of psychological or emotional stress through physical symptoms) causes pains and cramps. In return, the brain receives two simultaneous negative messages that it will have to process: 1) I have been dismissed from my job, and this means I'm not good enough; and 2) my stomach hurts, which means I am sick. These two pieces of information connect and intertwine in a particular part of the brain, and set off depressive symptoms. By treating the stomach first (through therapy such as non-invasive Visceral Manipulation), we can eliminate the conflict the person was processing in the organ. The brain then perceives a positive change, and the person, freed of pain, has a better chance of solving the job-loss problem.

Recurrent stomach pains can cause anxiety—notably the fear of being permanently affected and developing a more serious ailment. In the unconscious mind, the threat of cancer begins to loom. We all have a tendency to imagine the worst possible scenario. This kind of worry does not encourage us to try to adapt or solve a conflict at work. Helping an organ to function better allows the person to feel more confident.

Healing an Organ by Treating an Emotional Problem

Sometimes an organ can remain deaf to any treatment, allopathic or naturopathic. The problem turns out to be essentially psychological. In such cases, specific treatment is necessary. The practitioner can advise the patient to see a psychotherapist who will help him or her understand the causes of the physical discomfort. By learning to know yourself better, you can explore the meanderings of your psychological makeup and its somatic repercussions. That is what we are going to focus on throughout this book:

- What is at the origin of the problem, the organ or the emotion?
- Which of the two should be given priority?

The following pages will explain the specific physical, nutritional, and psychological requirements of each organ in order for it to remain in good health.

What If an Organ Has Been Removed?

When removing an organ, do we remove the emotions that are linked to it? This question may seem preposterous, in many ways. But nonetheless, it deserves careful attention. Every organ is connected to the brain, via a complex system of nerves, and sometimes hormones. The brain and the organ are in permanent connection. Removing an organ does not remove the representation of that organ in the brain. A person who has undergone an ablation can still produce psychosomatic reactions, transferred to another organ. If the gallbladder has been removed, the stomach may take over, and react psychosomatically to emotions. In any case, negative influx will always find a way to express itself and be evacuated. We have seen that the body is laced with 62,000 miles of nerves (again, two and a half times around the Earth!), which are attached to the spinal cord and to the brain. They keep the brain informed of everything that goes on in the body. How do we perceive the surgical removal of an organ, and how does our body perceive it? As a favor to our health, since the organ had become a danger to us. But the question is, why did this organ develop a major problem in the first place, making it necessary to operate. Why, for example, did the removed gallbladder produce gallstones? For the person who was operated on, it may be useful to find an answer to this question. Surgery may have solved the consequences of the problem (which is a good thing in itself), but did not necessarily discover the cause. Science cuts up bodies with a scalpel. Surgery is hyper-specialized. But the functioning of the body, from head to feet, is one, indivisible, process, a chain of linked mechanisms that vibrate in unison. The body reacts to every aggression, and always demands explanations. In-depth answers are not always to be found in the part of the body that experienced the pain.

PART TWO

What Your Organs Think

The "Organic Person"

As we have seen, each organ is connected to specific emotions. It is important to pinpoint the psycho-emotional discomfort associated with each organ and the disturbances it can set off. All the portraits in this book are empirical (based on experience) and include all the character traits that might be altered by dysfunction of the given organ. Not all the symptoms are necessarily present in one individual. When the physical problem improves, the person's behavioral stability returns, to a greater or lesser degree. But the tendencies pertaining to his or her weak link will remain and arise again if the organ encounters a new problem.

Take the case of a person who has trouble defining and finding himself. He belongs to the psycho-emotional "liver" type. His liver is a weak link in his body. If his liver starts causing problems, the psychological tendency linked to this organ will inevitably be accentuated. We all show signs of each tendency at different times. Sometimes, we are surprised by our own behavior. Let's say you're basically a generous person, but sometimes, for no apparent reason, you suddenly act stingy. This kind of change in behavior is no coincidence. It is caused by passing psychological tensions and visceral dysfunction, particularly of the intestines.

This book was not written to cast judgment upon ourselves or others. It simply notes facts and establishes causal relations. It helps us understand how we—and others—function as a whole, body and mind. For example, a person whose stomach gives her trouble will be better equipped after reading the book to understand her symptoms and find the right solutions. Her family and friends will also benefit from this knowledge. Understanding the mechanisms and modifications of our behavior and how they relate to a dysfunctional organ can help us deal with our problems more efficiently.

Now it is time to get acquainted with the "thinker" in our body: the brain.

5

The Brain: The Big Boss

The brain is a tribute to ingenuity. With all its complex architecture, it is uncannily similar to that of a walnut. To give you some statistics: it weighs 2.8 pounds, or two percent of our total body weight; it uses twenty percent of the oxygen in our body; and it consumes sixty percent of an adult's supply of carbohydrates (seventy-five percent of a child's).

How the Brain Works

The brain appears to be in perpetual motion. It developed as the animal world evolved. The primal brain of the very first humans was all instinct and emotions. Later on, as we evolved, the brain wrapped itself in thought-endowed gray matter, capable of speech and reason, of absorbing facts and solving complex problems. The results of recent studies show that at age twenty-one, the brain is not yet "finished": connections between neurons go on developing. That is to say that the human brain has not yet revealed all its secrets. More amazing yet, we do not feel the weight of the brain! Are we aware of this? No, but it is true. Indeed, the brain is kept afloat in the skull, in the cerebrospinal liquid, and thanks to the protective pressure of the skull, this brings its effective weight down from 2.8 pounds to 1.4 ounces.

The brain is the conductor in our great concert of emotions. It is the receptacle of everything that happens inside and outside us. It rules our emotions, relationships, metabolism, hormones, and nerves. It orchestrates and harmonizes our main bodily functions, such as digestion, movement coordination, and sexuality. It stores and sorts out the information it receives. (And, remember, it can pick up ten billion bits of information per second!) The brain thinks, therefore it builds: ideas, dreams, theories, theses....

It memorizes, and what a memory! It can keep the memory of a smell, a color, a gesture, a glance, something someone said, an impression, throughout an entire lifetime. Theoretically, it is the brain that decides when to take action. But sometimes the brain gets short-circuited by the body's nervous system, which can go into action faster than thought, or by emotional reactions which escape our conscious will.

Instinct and Reason

All acts commanded by reason transit through the brain. But when we're in danger, our instinct takes over and makes us react without the brain intervening. You are walking along a little country road. Right in front of you, a car misses a turn and falls into the ditch. Your self-preservation instinct can make you flee the place where the accident occurred, because you panic at the idea of a fire, an explosion, or of having to see wounded people. But little by little, reason takes over again. You go up to the car and offer help.

When it's all for the better. You often have to cross a certain road. That day, just like on so many other days, everything seems fine. Nothing coming from the left, nothing from the right. You are about to cross and you look straight ahead. Your brain has sent out its orders and you obey. Suddenly, instinctively, you jump back, and only at that point do you see the bicycle brushing by you. It was just about to knock you over. Your sensorial captors alerted you. A slight sound, an imperceptible movement, a dim presence or image—signals you didn't pick up a few seconds before—awakened your intuition to the imminent danger. Your nervous system instinctively saved you. It only informed the brain afterwards. At such moments, when our survival reflexes take over, a hundred million bits of information flood the brain simultaneously.

When it's all for the worse. During fires, you'll sometimes see "catastrophe scenes," or uncontrolled panic reactions—people may get trampled, or throw themselves out of a building's window rather than wait to be rescued. And unfortunately this does not usually come to a happy end. It would have been better if the victims had been able to see reason, rather than give in to panic. Let's imagine some less dramatic circumstances. You're invited to dinner, but you don't feel too great that evening. Tired out by a long day. The person sitting to your right at the table tries to start up a conversation with you, but you answer evasively and stick your nose into your plate. Obviously, you're doing nothing to try to be pleasant. In your tired state, a mere detail is enough to make the person seem off-putting to you. You lose all desire to make an effort and show any consideration. Maybe something in the person's looks or attitude reminds you of someone else you find unpleasant. In this case, your emotional and affective memory outdid your brain, which usually is the big boss. It let itself be overtaken! Too bad, maybe you missed out on meeting someone interesting. In other circumstances, in better shape, with less noise around you, less irritation, you might have enjoyed this person's company.

Right Brain, Left Brain: Theoretically, They Each Have Their Own Function

- The left brain's specialties include language (in right-handed people), calculation, logic, rationality, as well as positive and pleasant reactions such as joy or laughter.
- The right brain's field is hearing music, artistic creativity, intuition, imagination, and spatial orientation.

The brain records the emotions that most deeply affect our lives, and it is a fact that these are not usually the most pleasant ones. Sadness, melancholy, regret, remorse, frustration, and fear are all within its range. All negative! Because of this, the brain plays an important role in manifesting depressive symptoms.

It's largely in the parietal area of the right brain that powerful emotions settle, those that really mark you for life. Yet all parts of the human body are interdependent. Particularly in the brain, everything is connected: a total of one hundred million billion connections.

Photon and positron scans show that this right-side parietal area preserves the memory of our emotional past. It is not the only part of the brain that does so, but it is the most receptive. Fifteen years before these scanners existed, my hand had already located and felt this right-side parietal area in many of my patients. It is a real satisfaction to see that these perceptions have been verified by science. Official confirmation through medical imagery of what the hand feels is decisive in the course of evaluation and manual treatment. When a person shows signs of possible depression, specifically trained therapists are able to determine manually which part of the brain is involved, by feeling the cranium and detecting hyper-thermal areas.

Memory: An Amazing System

Before getting stored in the right-side parietal area, our memory of emotions goes through the limbic system, which is the most primitive part of our brain, made up of several small areas located within its deepest folds. This system processes and controls our emotions and the behavior they determine. We mustn't forget that emotion and instinct preceded thought. A hunting dog raised in an apartment very quickly recovers his hunting instinct as soon as he is let loose in the countryside. His ancestral genetic memory takes over. He naturally goes back to the original behavior of his breed.

Emotion, Instinct—What Is the Difference?

An emotion is a quick and intense, pleasant or unpleasant psychological reaction that acts mainly upon our organs.

Instinct is the way a specific species acts to ensure its survival and continuity. In everyday language, it can also mean acting impulsively, without thinking.

The Limbic System and the Organs: An Intimate Relationship

The limbic system is our emotional brain. It can react before the cognitive brain (which governs reason) has its say. The examples above clearly illustrate this distinction, such as the person who jumps out the window in panic.

In the limbic system:

- The amygdala controls the fear aroused in dangerous situations, or situations we perceive as dangerous. It rules our survival instinct. It receives emotional information and calls forth immediate, uncontrollable reactions, such as losing one's breath, cold sweat, panic, fleeing, fighting, etc.
- The hippocampus governs our learning processes. It is in charge of short-term memory (the memory of the immediate past).
- The thalamus is an indispensable sensory relay in the process of communication between organs, the body, and the brain.

When the Limbic System Isn't Working as well as It Should

The limbic system is the seat of many functions: breathing, heartbeat, libido, appetite, sleep, and hormonal stimulation, to name a few. It seems to be in command of a large portion of the body's physiological balance. But it is also the source of psychological disturbances such as anxiety or panic attacks. This is frequent in emotional people who are already overburdened, or people who have a very low reactivity threshold. This brings to mind the case of one of my patients, who had just become a widow and was going through a phase of heightened emotional sensitivity. She goes home at dusk. She passes a group of young people laughing and talking loudly. She steps up her pace. The group doesn't follow her, but nonetheless, when she reaches her doorstep and goes to put the key in the lock, she panics. She feels her chest constricting her as if she were caught in a stranglehold, her heart starts beating like mad, her hands shake and her knees go weak. A neighbor goes by just at that moment and notices that she is in trouble. The woman is leaning against the wall, she can barely breathe, and just manages to whisper, "Quick! An ambulance!" The neighbor immediately thinks of a heart attack and calls an ambulance to rush her to the hospital. Diagnosis: it wasn't a heart attack, even if it looked like one. It was a panic attack—the echo of an emotion in an organ! In fact, the limbic system had overpowered reason in this woman who was already distraught over the loss of her husband.

When we are in a highly emotional state, we lose our self-control, and therefore our ability to use reason. This is when our body experiences the immediate echo of these overpowering emotions. Our organs are the first to react, because they are intimately related to our limbic system. The connection is made by the thalamus. Visceral reflexes and instinctive behavior take over. These immediate reactions can be very powerful: a "knife" in the stomach, abdominal pain, vomiting, tachycardia, cramps, diarrhea, and others.

• Blackout: we shut off

When emotion overwhelms us, when it becomes intolerable, the emotional brain has an unfailing parry: it shuts off. Total short-circuit. No more pain, no more emotion, no more agitation. That is what we call "blackout." In other words, we "sync out." The brain uses this same process to fight unbearable pain. But syncope is only a very short-term solution: when the person comes to, the problems are still there, perhaps only slightly less intense: a bit of the "too-much" sometimes does get released in the process.

• Our body records everything

All primal reactions set off by the limbic system are unfailingly recorded in our organs. We can stifle the problem, bury it in the depths of our body, but it remains latent and can resurface. The symptoms may be less acute and less spectacular, but they can also be more severe: asthma attacks, a stomach ulcer, eczema, psoriasis, colitis or cystitis. Illness can also hook onto the body's weak link and appear later on. Under severe stress, bleeding recto-colitis that had never before manifested but was in the person's genes can suddenly develop. Sometimes, worse yet, a severe stress situation can be a triggering factor of cancer. Our immune system is very dependent on our emotional centers. Intense stress over a long period can weaken our defense system and generate or awaken serious illnesses.

How does the relationship between brain and organ function?

When a stress situation occurs, the brain gets the message in a more or less conscious way. However, the information can sometimes go directly to certain emotional centers, bypassing the conscious brain. This is often the case with fear, when the body reacts instantaneously, independently of your will: you suddenly steer sharply to the left, and then you realize that you actually did avoid a hole in the road or an animal. In such a situation, the brain reacts by sending nervous, chemical, and hormonal messages to the body. Sometimes the muscles are affected (tetany or trembling), but the organs are the main target. The organs react in turn and send back nervous, chemical, and hormonal messages to the brain. These messages can be instantaneous or deferred. For example, the pancreas can produce more insulin; the heart can start beating much faster (tachycardia) or irregularly (arrhythmia). The person can end up with recurrent tachycardia or arrhythmia. Visceral memorization takes its course: the organ's cells record the messages and send them back to the brain, immediately or later. These messages reinforce the emotional imbalance in the brain. It can therefore be said that the organ sets off an emotional resonance.

Indirectly, Our Organs Think!

There is a wavy line between the symptoms of a malfunctioning organ and one's emotional state. The brain doesn't always differentiate between what is physical and what is psychological, among the information it gets at the moment the stress occurs. This explains why an organ can be the source of a behavioral or emotional problem.

Let's look at the case of Stephanie, who is in the midst of a divorce. Things have not been going well with her husband. She regrets having to go through with the divorce and is unhappy about the situation. It means failure to her—the collapse of her whole life-structure and the end of a dream of spending a lifetime with her partner. "We got along so well," she says. At night, she is filled with remorse and can't sleep. She goes through it over and over again: "I should have…. He shouldn't have…. We should have…." Her nights are exhausting. She feels like her heart is being crushed and her brain wrung out. "My head is going to explode," she says. At dawn, she suffers from cramps in the right side of her stomach. She will find out later that it's the duodenum. The pain gets more and more frequent and intense. Her brain, which had been carrying the stress of the divorce for weeks, discharged part of it onto her duodenum, causing unbearable irritation and inflammation. In return, her duodenum bombards her brain with painful information, disturbing her sleep.

During the day, Stephanie sometimes feels that same abdominal pain, constantly reminding her of her psychological turmoil. It's a real game of ping-pong between her brain and her duodenum. Physical and psychological pain intermingle to such an extent that the brain cannot distinguish between them anymore. One reinforces the other and vice versa. You could say that her duodenum is also going through a divorce.

Male Emotions, Female Emotions

Men and women are not identical, emotionally speaking. They are different and complementary. It is a known fact that women are more prone to depression than men. The hormones (estrogen and progesterone) produced under the control of the pituitary gland and the hypothalamus apparently play a key role. This is thought to be proven by the mood swings that women go through at different phases of their cycle or during menopause. By the same token, it is recognized that men are more prone to violence, because of testosterone.

In addition to this, culturally speaking, men are still under the influence of the ancestral educational practice that even recently still made people say: "You mustn't cry, you're not a girl!" Such injunctions are as deeply anchored in our memory as slight physical trauma is rooted in our body. Here it is not the limbic system doing the recording, but the cerebral cortex, the part of the brain in charge of what we learn, of reason, and of emotional control. So this is serious stuff, well implanted in our brains!

Experiments with Photon Scanners

In 2005, I had the opportunity to work with Gail Wetzler, Physical Therapist, and Alain Croibier, Doctor of Osteopathy (two highly trained Manual Therapists), along with Dr. Daniel Amen, a research psychiatrist, in a study of the significance of manual therapy (specifically Visceral Manipulation) and its effects on the brain. Dr. Amen, author of *Change Your Brain, Change Your Life* and other books (based on more than twenty-five thousand studies of the brain), provided both pre- and post-treatment SPECT scan studies (single photon emission computed tomography) for our experiment. The SPECT measures cerebral blood flow and metabolic activity patterns in the brain. SPECT studies belong to a branch of medicine called nuclear medicine. The test uses a small amount of radioactively tagged compounds as tracking devices to show us which cells are most or least active and have the most or least blood flow.

The protocol consisted of eight patients with complex physical and psychoemotional pathologies. To get a baseline study, a SPECT scan was taken the day before our treatment and then immediately after our treatment for comparisons. Our treatment was based on Visceral Manipulation for the most sensitive organ or surrounding fascia found in each patient.

In every case, the brain reacted to the Visceral Manipulation treatment. The scanner recorded the changes in the limbic spheres, including the thalamus and proprioceptive centers. We were able to verify that the brain does not always distinguish between emotional and physical data. The potential barrier between the body and the brain—or between the physical and emotional factors—is not well defined. What is very clear is that the body and the mind function as one. The experiments demonstrated the fact that treating the organs can have an effect on our psychoemotional functioning.

How to Take Care of Your Brain

From a physical point of view

To keep your brain in good shape: breathe, be active, practice physical and mental exercise, read, count, memorize, go to the theater, go to the movies, join an association. Most of all, don't live an isolated life. It is generally accepted now that a person who keeps physically active is less at risk of developing Alzheimer's and related diseases. Physical exercise increases blood circulation and brings more oxygen and stimulation to the body's cells. Other chemical and hormonal factors activated through movement also play a role.

From a nutritional point of view

Your diet plays a major role in the health of the brain, as the brain is the greatest glucose consumer in our body. To ensure that you are feeding your brain what it needs most, include a healthy dose of complex carbohydrates in your daily intake. Athletes, who need a lot of it to achieve the best possible performances from their body and muscles, are not always aware that complex carbohydrates are so necessary for the brain. They are good for the body and the mind.

From a psychological point of view

Take care of your mental state: yoga, relaxation, and positive thinking are all beneficial mental exercise (if guided by competent teachers) to help us remain active and to keep on enjoying life. It is useful to learn how to tame one's emotions without blocking or diverting them. If things seem to have gone off track in your head, don't hesitate to turn to therapists—homeopaths, acupuncturists, manual therapists, relaxation therapists (see page 224)—who will help you bring your brain and organs back into balance. If you really can't solve the problem, try a psychotherapist or a psychiatrist.

There is no such thing as a sane mind without a healthy body. This is nothing new, as illustrated by the Latin phrase *"Mens sana in corpore sano,"* meaning "a healthy mind in a healthy body." But there is also no such thing as a healthy body without a healthy mind. We never forget a painful event; we learn to accept and integrate events in our life and evolution. The pain of losing a loved one will never be erased. Even if it loses some of its edge, it will stay rooted in our fibers forever. We have to acknowledge this fact: "I am still alive, life goes on, I have to accept this death in order to restore my own balance and harmony." So why not put energy into perpetuating the thoughts and acts of the departed person? Act in her memory, honor his values. Relive his or her positive perceptions in the small details of daily life. For example, "He (or she) loved the sea (or the mountains), so I'll look at them with twice as much pleasure or intensity."

6

The Lungs and the Bronchial Passages: A Lot of Wind, or Just a Breeze

The lungs are so precious that they are wrapped up in the pleura (a double-layered membrane) and totally protected by the rib cage. They are the organ of breath. One speaks of "the breath of life." This breath can be heard. Think of the tender image of a mother leaning over her baby's cradle to hear it breathe. The respiratory rhythm consists of fourteen breathing-in/breathing-out cycles per minute, about six hundred million times in a lifetime. The air we take into our lungs, along with the food we put into our digestive system, is the fuel for our vital energy.

We are often told, and rightly so, to take a "deep breath of fresh air." Indeed, our health depends on the quality of the air we breathe. The air reaches the lungs via the bronchial tubes and feeds oxygen to our blood. The blood goes into the pulmonary artery to circulate to the rest of the body, and the out-breath carries the carbon dioxide that is a waste product of the body's metabolism. The lungs and the bronchial tubes, along with the nose and the windpipe, are our first defenses against noxious factors in the air, such as pollution.

How the Respiratory System Works

From Water to Air

In the womb and at the moment of birth, a baby's lungs are filled with water. As we know, it is only once the umbilical cord has been cut and the baby exposed to air that the lungs fill up with air. At that very moment,

41

the child screams. He has just begun his earthly life, with its reflex cycle of breathing in and breathing out. This transformation of the lungs, from "full of water" to "full of air," seems to be the explanation for the link that has been established between the lungs and fear of suffocating or drowning.

The Pleura's Role

The pleura is a double-layered thin membrane. One layer covers the lungs and the other lines the inside of the chest wall that cushions the lungs. The pleura's two layers offer the lungs tight-knit protection. There are only a few airtight tenths of an inch between the two, a fine layer of void that allows the lungs to move without rubbing. The pleura normally releases a small amount of fluid. The fluid helps the lungs move freely during breathing. All the organs in our body are in perpetual movement. Like the parts of a motor, organs need lubrication to avoid overheating. Without any lubricant between the pleura and the lungs, the pleura would become irritated and produce excess pleural fluid, which could stagnate and seriously compress the lungs. Breathing would require much too much energy, and the person would be in danger of suffocating.

As with the heart, the walls of the pleura need to be perfectly smooth, both on the inside and the outside. Its two layers are as smooth as porcelain, so they can glide against each other without bumping. This way, breathing is easy and demands very little energy. Imagine a piece of soap sliding over a slightly damp marble surface. Between the two layers, the pressure is negative; this maintains the lungs in a state of dilation and helps the heart pump blood from the veins. To remain in optimal functioning condition, the pleura must protect itself from smoke, dust, coal, certain chemical substances such as asbestos, and generally speaking from all polluting agents. Physical trauma to the spine and the ribs can make the pleura sensitive and therefore, should be treated.

Do We Breathe Only Oxygen?

We tend to think that we inhale only oxygen. This is wrong. In fact we inhale seventy-nine percent nitrogen and twenty-one percent oxygen, along with water vapor and a few rare gasses such as helium. But oxygen is indispensable to all the cells in our body, and the entire twenty-one percent we absorb gets used.

Our Lungs, A Means of Communication with the Outside

Every day, we breathe in and out about twenty-one thousand times, and approximately twenty-four hundred gallons of air go in and out of our lungs daily—more than enough to fill a water tank! The medulla oblongata, located just above the spinal cord, orchestrates the respiratory cycle by activating the diaphragm. This muscle contracts, allowing the thorax to modify its volume during inspiration and expiration. The movement of breathing is automatic, but our brain can impose its will. While we have no power to control our heart directly, we can learn to control our breathing perfectly well. The most exceptional examples of this are yogis and deep-sea divers, who can hold their breath for more than five minutes, which is absolutely unthinkable for the average individual. However, anyone can practice breathing, relaxation, and yoga techniques that help us let go of tensions in the body and the mind.

How to Breathe Better

- Lie down on your back, legs bent, arms slightly outspread, palms turned upwards. Place a very light cushion on your stomach and breathe in, pushing the cushion upwards, then breathe out tucking your stomach in, with the cushion following the movement.
- Start with short, rather quick breathing cycles, and end with slow, ample breaths. Practice for two minutes every day.
- Still lying on your back, in the same position, try to press your entire body, one part after the next, onto the floor, going from the head down to the feet. You should feel your body and its heat resting on the floor. Take particular care with the small of the neck and the pelvis, which will tend to resist. Practice this exercise once a week, twenty times in a

row. The pleura attaches directly to the cervical spine, and its
movement is dependent on tension levels in the abdominal
and pelvic cavities. This exercise will decrease those tension
levels; this has a direct effect on the ability of the pleura to
move freely, particularly where it attaches at the cervical
spine.

The carbon dioxide content in the blood can modify our breathing. An
abnormal increase of carbon dioxide can cause suffocation. The lungs
and the kidneys are the key elements in homeostasis (the body's internal
balance). Together they regulate the acidity level in the body, the famous
pH. Compare this to a swimming pool: if the pH level is wrong, nothing works anymore—the water isn't clear, the bottom of the pool gets
filled with algae, the filters are obstructed. Too much CO_2 disturbs the
body's main functions, and first and foremost its acidity level, its pH. This
causes dysfunction. The kidneys get blocked, the heart beats too rapidly,
muscles are tetanized. Nothing works anymore!

The lungs also protect the body from pathogenic agents. They are the
antechamber of immunity. From the right side of the heart, the lungs
receive dark-red venous blood, poor in oxygen and rich in carbon dioxide. They return the same blood, now crimson red, to the left side of the
heart, rid of its carbon dioxide and enriched with oxygen.

The Bronchial Passages, an Exchange System

The numerous branches of the bronchial passages, from the bronchi-
oles to the pulmonary alveoli (we have close to three hundred million
of them), allow the air to circulate in the lungs. Every day they produce
one quart of secretions to moisten the lungs and evacuate impurities.
This liquid spills directly into the digestive tube. That is why we don't
even notice it, except when we have a cold or congestion. In that case, we
get rid of the excess secretions by coughing and spitting them out. The
bronchial tubes are covered with little cilia (hairs) that carry along the secretions and impurities—a conveyor belt for waste matter. All polluting
agents go through this process, in particular tobacco.

When the Lungs Don't Work as well as They Should

Before talking about dysfunction of the bronchial tubes and the lungs, we have to take a look at their worst enemy.

• Tobacco: the number-one enemy

It's written big and bold on cigarette packs, and it's true. Tobacco is a threat to life. It attacks the respiratory system first, since smoke goes into the body through the respiratory tract. Tobacco increases bronchial secretions, but most of all, it anaesthetizes the cilia that line the bronchial tubes. Deprived of their "conveyor belt," the bronchial passages can no longer do their job of carrying out waste. The secretions stagnate and can become infected. One unpleasant consequence: the smoker starts coughing up yellow mucus. This is a bad sign, but the problems don't stop there. Little by little, the diameter of the bronchial tubes decreases. Pressure in the lungs increases. The air can't get through properly anymore, and breathing becomes difficult. There is a whistling sound. The blood no longer receives its normal oxygen supply, and the entire organism suffers from this. Today, lung specialists believe that smokers face a forty times higher risk of developing cancer than do non-smokers.

About Passive Smoking

This is an element that should be taken into consideration more often: when you're talking about a smoke-filled room, passive smokers are not all equal. Weight plays a determining role—the lighter you are, the more your body will be intoxicated. Let's take, for instance, a hundred-and-fifty-pound person and a seven-pound baby. The intoxication factor is at least twenty-three times greater for the baby.

It is believed that a passive smoker absorbs about half the smoke exhaled by smokers. Be aware of this. Never bring babies and children into a smoking area!

• When breathing becomes difficult

When the respiratory system isn't working well, the first "penalty" is that it becomes difficult to breathe normally. Breathing in and out can become noisy. Fatigue, lack of energy, and backache in the shoulder blade area are symptoms of a breathing deficiency. Untimely bouts of aggressiveness can be explained by the presence of excess carbon dioxide in the blood. The person runs out of breath at the slightest effort. The heartbeat accelerates, the pulse quickens. The person gets pains in the side. Excessive sweating can also be a sign of breathing difficulty. The skin isn't as pink, with the change in color especially noticeable under the nails, which become bluish-gray. Be careful—if you start coughing too much or in an unusual way (a dry cough, coughing up a lot of phlegm), go see your doctor. A person who is breathing poorly puts a lot of stress on his or her body, and develops poor posture.

• When breathing becomes noisy

For one of my building projects, a team of architects was hired, and we had several meetings with the various people working on the project. Among them was an industrial draftsman who always stayed in the background and acted more like someone who just carries out orders than a creative professional, asserting his ideas. And yet his rare comments, expressed with difficulty in chopped-up phrases, were full of common sense and always added something to the discussion and the work project. Leaning over his draftsman's desk, he seemed to lean into it more and more with every breath. He breathed noisily and seemed ill at ease. Whenever I happened to be alone with him, he would share his ideas more freely and speak more fluidly. I sensed in him a constant desire to fade into the background, despite the high quality of his work. Later on, this man came to me as a patient and told me a lot about himself. He had had tuberculosis at age fifteen, and had suffered from respiratory failure ever since. This recurrent problem had determined his respiratory behavior and his attitude at work.

"It's terrible," he told me. "At meetings when everyone is being quiet, the only sound in the room is my breathing. At such moments, I feel like disappearing from the room. It is so hard to have to impose one's physiological problems on a whole assembly." This man felt locked up inside a cage—his rib cage! After a few sessions of re-education and respiratory positioning with a physical therapist, this man learned which postures helped him breathe better, with more ease and freedom.

• *Our emotions can upset our respiratory rhythm*

We have all at some point in our life experienced an emotion that made us pant or stop breathing for a moment. These are reactions commanded by our emotional brain, in particular by the thalamus and the limbic system. But we have the means to restore our normal breathing rhythm: by breathing deeply, slowly, and concentrating on the in-and-out movement of our chest, we can quiet down our breathing. It is much more difficult to intervene in an emergency, when the heartbeat goes haywire. You have to contact a doctor immediately.

~Lung–Bronchial Passage People~

We can hide certain kinds of organ dysfunction. But this is much more difficult when it involves the lungs. A respiratory problem is easily noticeable. It can be seen in the person's posture, the color of their skin, their sweatiness. You can hear the noise their breath makes. It is raucous, whistling, labored.

• *Too much or not enough*

"Lung people," or people whose weak link shows up in the lungs, often have an ambiguous attitude. They go from too much to not enough; they defy the classic notions of a balanced character. Understandable: the imbalance is in them, since their "fan" doesn't always function properly!

"Not enough": Lung people can seem shy, subdued, almost fearful. They walk at a slow pace, hiding in their shoulders. They are a long way from the frame of mind and the attitude of a winner. Add on to this a feeling of being locked in, as well as various inhibitions. They are afraid to bother people and have a tendency to stand back. They can do very well, but their lack of self-confidence hampers their intentions. So they tend to

live out their wishes in their dreams. They can be claustrophobic, agoraphobic, hypochondriacs. Phobias are part of their daily life. A lung person with respiratory problems constricts his or her vital space even more.

"Too much": Some lung people have a very stiff posture. They often take up too much space, to the point of not letting others express themselves and bloom in their presence. These lung people want to rule like a sovereign and cannot stand being contradicted. They set up challenges for themselves, to impose their personalities even more upon others. And yet, they often go against their own nature in doing so. After all, authority might not be their strongest point! They may put on an independent front but actually display a clear need for emotional support. Behind their show of vigor and dominance, a certain weakness may be detected.

André, the head of a small company, has asthma attacks that come in cycles. When his breathing is OK, he leads his team dynamically, takes constructive initiatives, and never doubts the accuracy of his decisions. When he is going through an attack, he gives up and becomes pessimistic. His partner takes over and manages the company. André leaves everything up to him, and lets himself be guided. At such times, he even tends to slow down the company's business. He goes from the attitude of a lion to that of a mouse. He knows it, but his illness often overpowers his will.

Whether acting along the "too much" or the "not enough" lines, the difficulties that lung people have to face are the same, as we will now see.

• Poor management of their own territory

Everyone needs to find their place and "fill their own space," in relation to themselves and to others. This doesn't normally imply any desire to dominate or be aggressive toward other people, or to encroach upon their territory. If you don't naturally occupy your own territory, you risk being invaded by others, and most of all, you're not letting your own personality bloom.

• Lack of self-confidence

Nobody is totally and continuously self-confident. We all have ups and downs. But a recurrent lack of self-confidence is harmful to the development of one's personality. Most of the time, difficulties in occupying one's own territory are linked to a lack of self-assurance. Respiratory problems cost so much energy that the ailing person doesn't have the strength to dare anymore. He or she loses confidence. This attitude is even more pronounced when the person was educated in an atmosphere filled with negative messages, real or implied, such as: "Don't do that, you won't be able to" or "Go away, this isn't your place here."

• Domination and fear of being dominated

Lung types show a certain admiration toward people who dominate them. Paradoxically, they are terrified by the idea of being taken over, dominated by an individual or group. When dominated, they feel like they are suffocating! This is a real dilemma for people who don't always know how to find their place and protect their territory. *Horror vacui—* Nature abhors a vacuum"—this old adage implies that the place we leave empty will no doubt be taken by somebody else very soon!

Conversely, the lung person can sometimes be the dominant one. Pushing their chest forward, they like to show that they "pack a punch," and they impose their point of view and ideas forcefully. Yet you sometimes get the impression that it would take very little for that chest to deflate and for the person to lose his "big airs."

• Fear of confrontation

Lung people feel uncomfortable when they have to confront difficult people or face conflict situations. They tend to elude or disregard them. Sometimes they will confront someone or try to solve an impossible problem, but more often than not their effort is futile. Jean-Claude, who suffers from respiratory deficiencies—only has occasional attacks, but they tire him out and limit his field of action. Every year, he has to choose a place to go on vacation with his wife. They never agree, and they fight over it. Because of his respiratory problem, Jean-Claude doesn't like heat or humidity, whereas his wife dreams of beaches and palm trees in the tropics. "I've noticed that when I'm in good shape, I can stand up for my choice, but when I'm having trouble breathing, I become passive. For instance, this year we're going to Djerba [a Tunisian island]—not the ideal place for me, you know!" he concludes.

• *Withdrawal*

Withdrawal occurs when someone feels out of place, permits others to dominate him or her, avoids confrontation, and remains passive. Having been through too many situations that made them feel uncomfortable, they withdraw into themselves. It's the snail syndrome. They go back into their shell! They build themselves a tiny little shelter where they feel protected.

• *Fear of bothering people*

This attitude is a companion and partial result of many of the previously mentioned traits of lung people who are experiencing respiratory difficulty and feel fragile: they become chronically fearful. But it is hard to tell if this shyness is merely a result of their poor respiratory functioning or if other factors, such as education or character, are the greater influence.

• *Dependency*

Lung people need the support of a strong (or at least seemingly strong) person to feel reassured. They use this person as a tutor, a guide, a catalyst. They lack breath and therefore stamina to go ahead on their own. This is the case with François, who suffers from chronic bronchitis. When he is going through a bout of it, he's very short of breath and gets exhausted quickly. Just doing his daily shopping becomes a problem. He says that his sister is the only person who can help him feel stronger.

"When I don't feel well, I can't help it—I just have to call my sister. She reassures me, shakes me up a bit and gives me courage. When I'm OK, she rarely hears from me," François admits. "She doesn't complain about it—that's how our relationship works."

Respiratory function is very much affected by a number of environmental variables: cold, heat, humidity, and altitude, to name a few. It's an ordeal for the sensitive person but also for the people around him or her, who often become subject to these circumstances and conditions.

• Lack of authority

Authority can be exercised naturally, by virtue of the position we occupy, or both. A lung person who has real respiratory problems and/or a sensitive constitution would like to show authority but doesn't always know how to. It is true that the attitudes described here are not conducive to asserting oneself. We could call it "lack of punch."

• Claustrophobia and its opposite

It may seem contradictory for a person whose tendency is withdrawal to suffer from a phobia of closed-in or crowded spaces. In fact, it is one of the paradoxes of lung people. Because they don't breathe efficiently and don't feel well, they close up. But once inside their shell, they feel the need for open spaces, where they think they might find all the air they need to breathe better. This tendency to withdraw or "shut oneself in" actually maintains respiratory distress.

One patient confided to me: "When I'm not feeling too well, I dream of being in a little cabin in the middle of a vast, open space, with the door open." This thought really illustrates the lung person's paradox: wanting to open up and close up at the same time.

A similar dynamic occurs with water—the lung person feels both attracted and afraid. Being afraid of water actually means being afraid of lacking air. For example, Antoine, who loves the sea and is an excellent swimmer, contracted a light case of tuberculosis at age twenty-five. Ever since then, he has been afraid of the water and doesn't dare swim long distances in the sea the way he used to do.

• Fear of suffocating or drowning

This fear is probably related to the way the lungs and the bronchial passages work. In the womb, the baby's lungs are full of water, and at the moment of birth they fill with air. If this transition occurs in difficult conditions at birth, the baby probably experiences fear of suffocating. Later on, this person will suffer in any situation where he or she may perceive a lack of air: swimming or scuba diving, for example. Fear can be provoked by chronic stress or sudden alarm and by any condition of constriction—for example, if someone is oppressing them (physically or otherwise), or even if their clothes are felt to be too tight. This fear of suffocating or drowning does not have to be precipitated by a birth trauma, though it is a common underlying cause. A lung person is predisposed to this phobia because of the weakened state of the lungs.

• Aggressiveness and hostility

As mentioned at the beginning of this section, excess carbon dioxide in the blood makes people involuntarily aggressive. The feeling of not being able to breathe properly can cause such a reaction. This aggressiveness can manifest itself verbally as well as physically. Here's another example from among my patients—a very nice young man, Marc is an asthmatic. But when he is going through a bad asthma attack, he can suddenly turn violent, which is out of character for him. Once, for no apparent reason, he punched a young physical therapist who was working with him on respiratory reeducation. The impulse came from his dis-ease and feelings of injustice and powerlessness that sometimes arise in him when faced with people who have no trouble breathing—like this physical therapy practitioner, who was young and in excellent shape. For Marc, it was a feeling of hostility that comes from deep in the marrow!

•Helpfulness

Although lung people may have bouts of aggressiveness, they can also be helpful, devoted, and generous when they're feeling well. It's a way of thanking those who were there for them when the lung person felt unwell and needed help or comforting.

• A need for affection and attention

"I need other people's affection. I must get it, even if it means dramatizing my breathing problems a little bit to get the attention of people around me," confesses Jérémie. His behavior cannot be considered emotional blackmail because of his very real respiratory disease; however, it does come pretty close. A physical handicap often leads to a greater need for warmth, emotional presence, and understanding. Lung people have a tendency to complain in order to be pampered and to gain people's affection. It's a rather childish attitude, but it works almost a hundred percent of the time—for adults as well as children! Scold a child, and he or she might try to alarm you by coughing loudly, making you think he's about to suffocate!

• Suppressed feelings

As we've emphasized, the thorax is a chest (in both meanings of the word) containing precious treasures: the heart and the lungs. A treasure chest is meant to be locked. Lung people can be said to act like a chest because they are "closed" and very good at not saying things. When they speak of love, it is through the eyes, rarely with words or by quoting a poem. The husband of an asthmatic woman shares, "I have to fish for tender words from my wife."

• Rigidity

Lung people are sometimes paradoxical: they can be rigid in their intimate circle, where they don't feel shy, and quite malleable outside this circle, in a professional or social context. They are full of principles that they try to transmit to those around them. The bars of the cage they lock themselves in are often very rigid.

• Childhood fears are still present

Childhood fears were necessary for us to build our personality. They survive in our unconscious mind and reappear in particularly stressful situations. Lung people bring these old fears to the surface somewhat regularly, and might even describe them as their constant companions. Such people say things like: "It's ridiculous to be afraid of the dark or of ghosts, but I can't help it."

Mireille has just been through a very severe attack of asthma that left her totally drained. When she describes the most difficult moments of the attack, she says that in the moment she remembered playing hide-and-seek as a child: "I was always terrified that someone would suddenly find me and frighten me. I used to close my eyes so I wouldn't have to see the danger I felt was imminent. Even now, when I get an asthma attack, I sometimes feel the same thing."

• From fatalism to rebellion

Asthmatic people have to accept the fact that they will experience attacks. One has to face them and wait for them to pass. Often people end up resigning themselves to it. Exclamations such as "It just had to happen" or "There's nothing to do about it" are daily fare with lung people. Sometimes they rebel against the injustice of it: the simple act of breathing is a problem for them, and it just doesn't seem fair to have to struggle with such a basic act of survival.

• A vivid imagination

What could be better than the imaginary world to escape reality? The stronger the pressure, the more vivid the imagination. Just by looking at a postcard, a lung person can describe Hawaii to you or take you on a wild adventure in the Galapagos.

How to Take Care of the Lungs

From a physical point of view

How not to lack air? It is possible to recover your lung energy—with exercise, exercise, and more exercise. Remember that we breathe because of our rib cage's capacity to change its volume. The pleura, the envelope surrounding the lungs, is made up of two membranes that slide over each other. Between them, there is that negative pressure that allows the lungs to fill up with air. To be able to fulfill its function, the pleura has to be supple and distensible. Therefore, any exercise that expands the thorax and stretches the arms is welcome.

But what exercises?

- To stimulate the heart and breathing, nothing is better than walking, or better yet, quick walking, cross-country running, bicycle riding, swimming, and stretching. Do it at least once a week, for two hours.

- Stretching along the entire spine, chest, and rib cage will increase the space within which the lungs can freely move.

- To help make the pleura more supple, you can try hanging from a bar, but do it progressively. At the beginning, keep your feet resting on a stool; only try without the stool once you feel perfectly at ease with the stretch. This exercise is also very good for your arms and ribs (to which the pleura is attached). Take a few minutes to give yourself a massage between your ribs every now and then.

- Learning to control your breath will guarantee you better health. Work on holding your breath briefly, on breathing in and out quickly, on panting. You may have some experience already if you practice yoga or relaxation, or if you are a woman and you took childbirth classes.

- If you're having a hard time re-educating your breathing on your own, do it with a manual therapist or join a yoga or relaxation class. Start exercising gently. Don't put yourself under any pressure—this would only increase the anxiety linked to your respiratory problems.

A Few Stretching Exercises

The following movements help stretch the spine, the ribs, and the pleura.

- Standing, in profile, one arm stretched up against a wall, your feet at a slight distance from the wall, try to stretch the other arm as far as possible upwards, while pushing your thorax against the wall. Repeat this movement about twenty times with each arm, once a day.

- Standing, hands linked behind your neck, leaning against a wall or a door, breathe in deeply, pushing your elbows toward the back, and breathe out loosening the position slightly. Repeat the movement about thirty times a day.

- Intercostal (between the ribs) stretching is excellent for you: lie on your back, your arms spread out and knees bent. Slowly move both knees to the left and then to the right, as close to the floor as possible, keeping the arms on the floor. Do this about twenty times, once a day.

A few more maintenance tips:

- Stop smoking. I may be repeating myself, but this is crucial. It is better to be alarmist than permissive. Tobacco kills people young, with intense suffering!
- Avoid polluted places: streets with a lot of traffic, smoky rooms, restaurants without ventilation or non-smoking areas. Also avoid hot and humid places.
- Beware of air conditioning, especially when it hasn't been used throughout the winter. Think of your car when summer comes around. Mold has formed and countless micro-organisms have been trapped in there for months— enough to attack your bronchial passages and cause a dry cough.
- Also beware of varnish and paint that can cause allergies.
- Spring air filled with pollen is often irritating for people with sensitive respiratory systems. In the event of severe allergies, it is advisable to wear a gauze mask to filter out dust and pollen.
- Have your spine checked. A single blockage point in one of the twenty-four ribs attached to the spine can impair the mobility of your rib cage and pleura.

From a nutritional point of view

- Avoid putting on weight. Excess weight will inevitably make the diaphragm and the lungs work harder. And remember that healthy breathing helps eliminate fat. So keep the whole process flowing.

- Avoid overburdening your liver. When the liver is clogged, all the mucous membranes get irritated and congested. Mucous membranes are found in many parts of the body—in the sinuses, bronchial tubes, stomach, intestines, and elsewhere. Most of all, beware of chocolate and alcohol, which can cause sinus infections or bronchitis in sensitive people. (For more on the liver, see the chapter dedicated to this organ, beginning on page 92.)

From a psychological point of view

We have seen that the lungs are involved where there is fear of suffocating, drowning, being locked up, and being oppressed or dominated. One can learn to negotiate one's fears and anxieties with the help of psychotherapy, relaxation, or yoga, depending on the severity of the psychological burdens.

7

The Heart: It Beats and Throbs

Located near the center of the chest and to the left, the heart is made up of a muscle called the myocardium, which encloses two distinct parts separated by the thick ventricular septum. Each half contains two cavities: the auricle and the ventricle. The right side sends de-oxygenated blood to the lungs, and the left side receives re-oxygenated blood back from the lungs. Blood always circulates in the same direction.

How It Works

A Very Powerful Pump

The heart is a small, ten-ounce machine that beats a hundred thousand times a day (the average cardiac rhythm is seventy beats per minute) and more than three billion times in a lifetime. Centenarians beat all records! Every day the heart expels the equivalent of 1,900 gallons of blood (the body contains about five quarts).

The heart is the first organ in the human body to begin functioning. By the time the embryo reaches its third week, its heart is already beating. And the heart is the last organ to stop functioning: when it stops beating, all bodily functions cease, and it's all over.

The first beats of a heart are somewhat of a miracle. A bunch of cells join together, and suddenly the heart quivers and then starts beating! This is the amazing spectacle of life coming into being. The heart beats, the blood circulates. If the blood were to rub against the walls of the heart, it would coagulate. That is why the inside of the heart is lined with a very smooth membrane called the endocardium. On the outside, the pericardium wraps the heart up inside two membranes separated by a fluid which protects it from any mechanical pressure. In this arrangement, the heart does not waste energy.

While the heart possesses its own command system and nervous system, its functioning can nonetheless be modified by the brain and the central nervous system. The cardiac rhythm is under the direct influence of our emotions, anxieties, and stress, any of which can make the heart beat very quickly (tachycardia) or in an irregular way (arrhythmia). Whenever the oxygen rate in the blood decreases, the heartbeat's rhythm increases. The quantity of oxygen or carbon dioxide in the blood, blood pressure, one's level of physical activity, body heat, as well as the intensity of stress or effort are among the data that the brain transmits to the heart, altering its rhythm.

A Cycle: Contraction—Relaxation

A contraction cycle lasts an average of four-fifths of a second. Under exertion or stress, it can go down to half that time. The contraction phase is called *systole* and the relaxation phase *diastole.* During the systole—in which the auricles contract first and then the ventricles in quick succession—the blood is expelled from the heart into the arteries to irrigate the entire circulatory system. During the diastole, the heart fills up with returning blood. The relaxation of the myocardium allows the blood to enter into the auricles and then the ventricles.

The *heart valves* control the flow of blood, opening and closing to the rhythm of the systoles and diastoles, in order to impede any blood reflux. Sometimes these valves are not as leak-proof as they should be and can cause heart murmur. In serious cases, this irregularity can tire out the heart muscle. Your doctor and his stethoscope are attentive to the slightest abnormal or unusual murmur. Luckily, small leaks are often of no importance.

The *pulse* indicates the rhythm of the cyclic contraction and release of the heart muscle. Usually the pulse is taken in the wrist. It is the expansion wave produced when the left ventricle contracts and this wave movement spreads through the arteries.

A Great Need for Oxygen

The heart's demand for oxygen is second only to the brain's. The coronary arteries bring the heart the oxygen it needs to function properly. "Coronary" derives from the word "crown." The coronaries surround the heart like a crown, feeding it about 95 gallons of blood per day, at rest. When the diameter of the coronary arteries is reduced by stenosis (narrowing caused by congenital or pathological sources) or cholesterol build-up, the heart lacks oxygen heightening the risk for heart attack. Tobacco, stress, hypertension (persistent high blood pressure), alcohol, and excess cholesterol are the coronaries' worst enemies. A cardiac muscle deprived of oxygen necroses. Cardiovascular danger is imminent!

When the Heart Doesn't Work as well as It Should

• Heartbeat disturbances

When we detect danger, our heartbeat speeds up, and it takes some time for it to return to its normal rhythm. Other emotions can also "quicken the pulse." Some people suffer from tachycardia (more or less permanent heartbeat acceleration); others from bradycardia (too slow a heartbeat). Highly trained athletes have a slow heartbeat, thanks to their increased ventricular capacity.

• Out of breath for no reason

Severe emotional stress, altitude, and over-exertion can be the cause of this type of disturbance. Sometimes circumstances seem insufficient to account for the acceleration of heartbeat and pulse. In this case, it is advisable to see your doctor.

• A tightness in the chest

This impression can be fleeting, can set in for a little while or, in rare cases, be felt for several hours. It happens spontaneously, and can be set off by an emotion. Nobody likes to feel tightness around the heart: we immediately imagine the worst possible scenario—especially men, who have the greatest risk of heart attacks. This tension is often due to tension in the heart's nervous system. Never hesitate to talk to your doctor about it.

• *Uneasiness in the chest*

This symptom can be recurrent. Sometimes it is felt when swallowing saliva or while eating. It feels like you're swallowing something too big.

• *Pain between the shoulder blades and down the left arm*

This is not a constant pain but one that comes and goes, usually on the left side with a tendency to radiate into the arm.

• *Pain in the jaws*

If such pain cannot be explained by mechanical dysfunction of the jaw (clenching of the jaws and grinding of the teeth during the night, for instance, or having chewed something too hard), it is advisable to see a doctor to discover the cause. The jaw muscles share some nerve fibers with the heart and the cervical vertebrae. This is how a heart problem can induce spasms in the jaws.

• *Pain in the neck*

As in the case of the left arm or the jaws, cervical (neck) pain can sometimes be caused by a heart problem. But this is rare.

• *A lasting stitch*

This is the same as the pain in the side we sometimes get after running too fast and/or for too long. The stitch can be felt on either side of the body. It comes and goes, depending on the activity we happen to be doing. It can even be felt in a resting position.

• *Sudden anguish*

Sudden, unprovoked anxiety can be a symptom of heart problems. Cold sweat and an uneasiness in the chest usually accompany this panicky emotion. It gives you the feeling of imminent danger. Usually, it's nothing. But do see a doctor.

> **• *Vertigo or a feeling of emptiness in the head***

A general feeling of floating, of no longer being attached to the ground, difficulty concentrating—these feelings can sometimes imply heart problems.

> **• *Extreme pallor***

Pallor or a pale cast to the face and skin, is due to a decrease in surface blood circulation. The body's priority is to ensure blood flow to the brain and heart. If this is insufficient, the body tries to block the blood flow toward other organs to divert more blood to the two neediest organs. The easiest and least dangerous place to take blood from is the skin. When the skin receives less blood, it turns pale. But the heart receives the benefit.

~Heart People~

Until we die, our heart never stops beating. If it is greatly affected by an emotion, it can go haywire at times. Love at first sight or sudden fear are familiar examples of something that can make our heart race. Joy, wonder, pride, shyness, and other emotions can be felt directly in the heart. There are many occasions where we can hear our heart beating. Sometimes it beats quite furiously! That is to say, emotions go straight to our heart!

> **• *The need to be loved***

Who can boast of not needing love? It is a universal need. To some people (particularly heart people), it is as important as the air they breathe. Their need to be loved is so strong that they are actually addicted to it. By wanting too much, they may end up being disappointed. "Love me!" they seem to be saying all the time. This need is usually addressed to their close circle. But sometimes they widen the circle of their demand to casual acquaintances. For example, some heart people can get very upset if a shopkeeper who is usually friendly suddenly seems indifferent toward them. This kind of reaction is typical of a strong addiction to love and affection.

• *Fear of not being loved*

Jacques was invited onto a research team—exactly the career he was aiming at. He went out of his way to be accepted by all the members of the team. Always being helpful, anticipating their wishes, offering to do odd jobs—and he actually went too far. Four members of the team started to find Jacques too clingy and began avoiding him.

Little by little, Jacques ended up being isolated from the rest of the group, without knowing why. "Look at everything I did for them!" he exclaimed. He couldn't analyze it himself, but his excessive need for recognition had turned against him. Jacques came to me because he felt a tightness in his chest, and all the objective medical tests were negative. As we worked together, I found a blockage in his back and ribs that created a constant twisting sensation in his thorax, causing the heaviness in his chest. While managing to ease the discomfort in his chest, I advised Jacques to start working with a psychotherapist to examine his fear of not being loved, so that this problem and its physical manifestations wouldn't become recurrent.

• *Excessive attachment*

In heart people, attachment to love borders on addiction to the loved one. This causes constant suffering whenever the other person seeks a bit of distance, goes away, considers separating, or finds another center of interest. As the original version of the French song "Chanson d'Automne" (Autumn Leaves) says: "Life separates those who love each other." This is often true, but it is particularly painful when one of the people involved is more dependent than the other.

• *The need for symbiosis*

If you seek symbiotic love or relationships, you take the risk of losing yourself, little by little, in the other person. That means forgetting one's own personality, to the point of putting oneself in danger. This transfer can sometimes be so strong that it impedes personal development. This need for symbiosis is often the result of too great an emotional demand.

• *Fear of being abandoned*

We all experience this fear when we feel betrayed or neglected by someone we love. But heart people tend to arouse and entertain this fear in
themselves, even when they have no sound reason to feel threatened.
With a malfunctioning heart, fear of being abandoned is particularly
strong. This fear is also related to other organs, such as the intestines and
the genital organs.

• *Jealousy*

There is a whole spectrum of jealous types, ranging from simple envy
to chronic jealousy in people who are jealous of their partner as well as
their friends. They become unbearable. Jealousy is like a deep-seated illness with them. They can only overcome it through psychotherapy or
psychoanalysis. Some people are jealous as a reaction to a clear and definite betrayal situation that they cannot bear. This form of jealousy often
is inevitable under such circumstances.

To give another example from among my patients: Francis has a whole
weekend to himself ahead. His wife is taking part in an advanced training
course in Paris. That is what she told him. He decides to go hiking near a
lake about an hour from their home. An extraordinary coincidence: from
afar, he sees his wife arm in arm with a man he doesn't know, but whom
she seems to know very well....

His reaction is instantaneous. He feels a burning in his chest. "Like being torn apart with a branding iron!" Francis said descriptively when he
came to see me. Ever since that fateful day, he has felt oppressed, physically and psychologically. Although medical tests show no injury to the
heart, the oppressed feeling is a direct consequence of that "stab" of jealousy experienced when he discovered his wife's betrayal. After several
treatments with Visceral Manipulation, the pain around the heart eased
up slightly, but the jealousy never went away. It lies latent and perks up at
the slightest little warning sign. "I never used to be jealous," Francis confided, "and now I get jealous over nothing. I've lost my bearings."

• Distrust

Heart people can move easily from total trust to distrust. Unmet emotional demands can bring on disappointment and suspicion. On the other hand, although they seem to distrust everyone, any smooth talker with a convincing line and oozing charm can win them over. An overly distrustful person can be easy prey for crafty people!

• Fear of judgment

Heart people have such a need to be loved that they have a hard time accepting any negative remark. To them, a negative opinion means that they are not liked, not loved, and that they are being ostracized.

• Generosity and the gift of oneself

Heart people are naturally generous. "She has a big heart!" people say. With their great need for recognition, you might be tempted to think that heart people only give to get in return, and to be appreciated. Acts of generosity can certainly stem from an emotional need. This can be seen when generous people are clearly disappointed when others don't recognize their generosity for its true value. "My whole life, I've been so devoted…" is a sentence you often hear. Certainly this is not always the case. Heart people can truly devote themselves for the sake of a cause.

• A certain form of narcissism

It is important to love oneself—this feeling is a solid base to build upon. But sometimes heart people have a bit too much self-love. To love oneself too much is dangerous, because the excess is often to the detriment of others.

• The need to be flattered and rewarded

Just as they love to be loved, heart people crave compliments and encouragement. They appreciate them under all circumstances, but even more so when they are given in front of other people. That is absolute happiness for them! You can do whatever you want with a heart person using flattery. Some women know exactly how to go about it with heart men. "Look!" one of them exclaims to her guests, "isn't our new garage beautiful? My husband built it." The husband turns pink with pleasure, and playing it down, says, "Oh, it was nothing, nothing, just a bit of work and patience."

• A tendency toward stage fright

Several organs are quite sensitive to stage fright, including the heart, the stomach, and the gallbladder. Stage fright experienced specifically in small groups, amidst people one knows or loves, is usually felt in the heart. That little congratulatory poem you have to read out loud to a friend on his birthday or the toast you plan to give at a wedding are typical examples of the type of situation that can make your heart beat faster than usual.

• Panache

We'll see in Chapter 11 that the stomach can be related to heroic acts. The heart is also involved in extraordinary actions that have a certain panache and flatter the ego. Heart people like to challenge themselves and test their own limits. They like to evaluate their performance in exceptional situations, under circumstances in which they can shine. There is a hint of narcissism in this type of behavior.

• Fear of manner of death

Being afraid of dying is not exactly the same thing as being afraid of death. Heart people are more worried about the manner of their death than about death itself. Obviously, death is unavoidable, but we observe that people die differently. Suffering and a long, slow decline can be more difficult to accept than the finality of death, especially for a heart person. A head of state of whom a journalist once asked, "Do you accept death?" answered, "Yes, but what I have a harder time accepting is not being alive anymore."

• Fear as a reaction

This is an immediate fear, in the face of a real or imagined danger. The heart starts beating so strongly that it seems to invade the whole thorax. We are not talking about deep-seated fear that develops over a long period of time, like the fear one encounters in kidney people (see Chapter 14). Instead, this reactive fear manifests in relation to an object, an event, or a hostile or dangerous situation. It is so strong that it cannot last for long: either it will be resolved and disappear, or it transfers the effects to other organs, such as the liver and the kidneys.

• Guilt

Guilt for a heart person applies to events connected with people they are close to. It comes about in situations involving a specific person—someone we were unable to help, a failed relationship, feelings that were inadequately expressed. It can also be the guilt felt after the death of a loved one, the remorse that makes us say: "I should have said that ... or done this ... I should have arrived sooner ... I should have been more present, offered more support or warmth...."

• Hatred

This type of feeling is no small matter, but fortunately it is rare. Since he was a child, Philippe always saw his father look down on his mother, treat her harshly, and denigrate her. His father's attitude toward his mother fueled a hatred in the son that grew with time. "When I was little, my dream was to grow very quickly so I would become stronger than my father and be able to stop him from hurting her. I even imagined fighting with him and beating him," Philippe explains. "When I crossed his path at home or elsewhere, my heart would start beating violently."

Philippe's father died of a heart attack at the age of thirty-five. Philippe hadn't grown enough to confront his father and get rid of his hatred. He was left with nothing but the memory of a destructive relationship, whereas he so badly wanted to be able to love his father. He felt as though his heart were caught in a stranglehold, the tightness pervasive. Psychotherapy made it possible for Philippe to free his heart to a certain extent.

• Rancor and remorse

Rancor and remorse, when related to burdensome problems, can affect the heart. In lighter cases, the problems move on to the gallbladder, and in the most severe cases, to the spleen. For more than a year, Béatrice—who was "in the pits" both emotionally and financially—had to leave her five-year-old daughter with her parents. Because of her job, she lived too far away to see her daughter regularly. In her own words, this situation "tore her heart apart." Throughout the period they were separated, she was consumed with remorse. Ever since, Béatrice has been suffering from serious cardiac arrhythmia.

• An incapacity to bear betrayal

Luckily, life more often puts us through small, recurring stress situations than through big, dramatic betrayal stories. Bernard, who owns his company, and Georges, his manager, have worked together for years. The company, which had been doing very well, begins to have serious problems. Fewer orders come in, and the competition gets fiercer and fiercer. Bernard tries to figure out what went wrong. He discovers that Georges had given most of their company secrets to their main competitor. Furthermore, Georges ends up quitting, only to be hired by the competition. Bernard was unable to bear Georges' betrayal—a man who not only had served as Bernard's "right arm" for years but was also a childhood friend. Bernard underwent triple bypass surgery in the months following these catastrophic (for him) events.

• Too great a pain

The pain and sorrow resulting from illness or the death of a loved one is felt as real, physical pain right in the heart. The heart literally tightens, feels heavy, and there can even be spasms. Some people immediately reach for their heart when they hear bad news. Of course, sorrow is not an emotion experienced exclusively by heart people, but since the heart is their weak link, it will be particularly affected.

• *Too powerful an emotion*

We all know this feeling—for instance, when we watch a very moving or sad film. Something tightens in our chest. Maybe we are trying not to cry. Usually this feeling fades rather quickly. But with hypersensitive people who tend to overreact, this pang can last longer, causing additional anxiety.

• *Distress*

Full-blown distress strikes when everything seems to be painted black, the suffering does not cease, and there appears to be no solution in view. The heart reacts first, then the pancreas and the spleen.

• *Joy, happiness*

An organ rarely manifests joy or happiness in an obvious way. When we are happy, the other organs simply do their job harmoniously. But the heart accelerates and starts knocking inside our chest: joy and happiness in rhythm!

How to Take Care of the Heart

It is vital to take care of your heart and keep it in good shape. Even if you smoke or have other health-damaging lifestyle habits, it is never too late to start limiting cardiovascular risk.

From a physical point of view

- *Train the muscle:* The heart is a muscle, and like any muscle it requires sustained activity to increase its strength and performance. Trained athletes have a slow heartbeat. Some professional cyclists have a cardiac rhythm of thirty-six heartbeats a minute (compared to the average person at seventy heartbeats a minute). Because its muscle power is increased, their heart propels a large quantity of blood with each contraction and therefore needs to work less. Exercise also optimizes the performance of the coronary vascular network. Even in cases where circulation is impaired, collateral circulation will develop and bring a better blood flow to the heart.

- *Stretch:* Stretch your thorax, because your heart needs to feel at ease inside the rib cage. Especially when the physical limitations of daily life (long periods spent sitting at work, for example) tend to make us tense up, we have to think about giving our heart space within our body by relaxing pericardial tensions. Stretching the thorax is beneficial to the pleura (the membrane surrounding the lungs) and the pericardial area (membrane around the heart).

  - If you work (or play) at a computer, avoid tensing up, slouching, and tightening your shoulders. Keep your glance horizontal, facing the screen, and your shoulders low and pulled back. This type of job makes it even more important to do stretching or tai chi chuan. If necessary, learn some appropriate stretching exercises from a physiotherapist or manual therapist.

  - *Favor progressive effort:* Choose activities that allow for a gradual increase in intensity or exertion. The heart is like a diesel motor—it doesn't appreciate or respond well to brutal, spontaneous effort; it needs to warm up first. Practice walking at a normal pace and then speeding up; cycle for several miles at a slower pace of pedaling; swim in lukewarm water; do cross-country skiing moderately in the beginning, without overdoing it. These are excellent activities for the heart. And most of all, don't forget that regularity always pays off!

  - *Take the time to warm up,* especially with sports that require quick bursts of energy or force, such as tennis or racquetball—these sports can be harmful to the heart if practiced without preparation. Run around the court a few times slowly, and do some stretching before you start to play.

- If you are a city dweller, do as much *walking* as possible. Avoid elevators, use the stairs, and if you can, go up a few extra flights.
- *Watch out for extremes and transitions.* If you have a slightly weak heart, beware of high altitudes, extreme temperatures (hot or cold), and sudden temperature changes. In summer, going from an air-conditioned room to very high outdoor temperatures can be a difficult adaptation to make.

From a nutritional point of view

- Follow the advice of a nutritionist to improve or fine-tune your diet for a healthy heart. (Remember that most doctors have very little training concerning diet.)
- Smoking is to be banned.
- Avoid cooked fats, excess sugar, alcohol, cold cuts, cream, ice cream, and salt (the latter contributes to high blood pressure). Check the sodium content of sodas, because they often contain a lot of salt. These foods are unhealthy for anyone, but particularly for people with heart problems.
- Eat as much soluble fiber as possible. This makes the liver slow down its cholesterol production, and therefore cholesterol rates are lowered generally in the body. Favor broccoli, cabbage, cauliflower, turnips, onions, leeks, carrots, lentils, white beans, watercress, and wheat germ; among the fruits, favor grapefruit, melon, peaches, apples, and prunes.
- Use olive oil, preferably of the highest quality: extra-virgin cold-pressed.
- Every now and then, add a few spoonfuls of canola oil to the olive oil, or dress your salads with walnut oil.

From a psychological point of view

Relax. Certain stress factors can be avoided. "Easy to say," you might answer, "but not easy to do." You must think about it and practice. When you are feeling tense, avoid confrontation. Learn to round your back. Yoga, relaxation, music, dance, and singing are all activities that can help you let go of your tensions. One of my patients, a fan of Jacques Brel (a popular singer in France), was able to lower her blood pressure two or three points just by listening to one of his records and singing along with him.

8

The Breasts:
Most Feminine of Symbols

A woman's breasts are a glandular organ. Their function is to produce maternal milk. They contain no muscle and are held in place by ligaments. Breasts are laced with a network of lymphatic vessels, connected to the lymphatic glands located in the armpits and at the base of the neck.

How They Work

Girls' breasts start growing at puberty (generally from the age of ten or eleven) under the influence of the estrogen produced by the ovaries. Women who generate too much estrogen have sensitive, sometimes even painful breasts, and they can have liver problems as well. This is because the liver eliminates estrogen and can become irritated when there is too much of it.

In general, the breasts are more sensitive during ovulation, which occurs from the twelfth to the fourteenth day of the menstrual cycle. In some women, the breasts are also more sensitive just before their period, between the twenty-fifth and the twenty-eighth day. The liver is particularly put to task during these periods of the cycle.

Breasts play an obvious key role in breast-feeding, and they also exert great attraction in a sexual context. Together with the pelvis, they are the image and symbol of femininity. A woman who feels at ease in her "woman's skin" stands up straight, with her chest forward.

When the Breasts Are Not as well as They Should Be

Women are usually well informed of the problems that the breasts can develop. But the deeper roots of these disturbances are to be found in hormonal dysfunction. The usual culprits are the pituitary gland, the hypothalamus, and the liver, which in turn are influenced by factors such as stress, eating habits, pollution, oral contraception and other hormone treatments, etc. Luckily, most women go for regular checkups and screening tests that can clear any suspicion very quickly. Listed below are some of the disturbances that can affect the breasts.

• Hypersensitivity

Breasts are usually most sensitive at ovulation (the fourteenth day) and just before the period (the twenty-eighth day). If this sensitivity evolves into pain during the period and especially throughout the cycle, it is an indication of hormonal imbalance.

• Congestion

The breasts seem larger and heavier. The slightest mechanical constraint or physical pressure leaves marks. Watch out for bras that are too tight.

• Lumps

The breasts are filled with fat tissue that can hide a tumor or give the impression that it is hiding one. That is why general practitioners and gynecologists perform a meticulous examination. Go for regular checkups.

• Discharge

Any discharge from the breasts not due to lactation is abnormal.

• Surface irregularities

If the skin on a breast looks drawn in, or if there are areas that look like small craters, you must see a doctor to ascertain the cause.

• When one breast is larger than the other

When the breasts are not the same size (more than just slight variances), from the time they develop on into adulthood, the cause is often scoliosis or a lateral imbalance of the thorax.

• Cervical or back pain

Certain nerves that end in the breasts come from the neck and back. Sometimes the breasts touch off pain in the spine, or vice versa. Some women with large breasts are uncomfortable walking or running, and may suffer from back pain. They will sometimes have their breasts surgically reduced in order to be able to move with more ease.

And what about men?

It is rare for a man to have breast problems. But let us note that at puberty or shortly before, a boy's breasts can grow slightly. This is due to a strong increase in estrogen at a time when the testosterone level is still low. This is often accompanied by weight gain. In such cases, the teenager is usually ashamed and hides under big sweaters or T-shirts. It is essential to reassure him and explain that everything will soon go back to normal—the weight as well as the breasts.

In mature men, such symptoms can indicate a problem with the pituitary gland. In the past, prostate problems were often treated with estrogens, which had a tendency to make the breasts grow in men. I saw male patients who were in despair over seeing this development in themselves. Such treatments are rare today and the dosages better regulated.

~Breast People~

Breast problems are a cry for help. Both men and women can be breast people; it is just more common for women and rare for men.

• *Recognizing her femininity*

During puberty, under the influence of estrogen, the little girl sees her breasts grow. She is becoming a woman. She can hide her pubic hair, but not her breasts. It is an important moment in the adolescent's life when she begins to display her femininity: the femininity she has, and the vision of the woman she would like to be and is simultaneously afraid of being.

• *The need to protect and be protected*

The tender image of a baby nursing at his or her mother's breast is a perfect symbol. The breast nourishes and protects. As a young mother said to me humorously, "When my child nurses, he is in my air bags." (She was referring to the image of cushioning and protective air bags in vehicles.) The breast woman wants to give this kind of protection, and she also wants to receive it from others. She is acting within the subtle "give and take" parameter.

• *Motherly love*

The breast is a potent symbol and reminder of maternal protection. Josiane always believed that her mother preferred her younger sister. Josiane's mother had always been very demanding toward the elder daughter, sometimes even harsh, and had never shown her much affection. Since her marriage, Josiane lived far from her mother and saw her infrequently. When she found out that her mother was dying, she rushed to her bedside.

"I absolutely want to see my mother before she dies, to hear her say she loves me!" Josiane lamented. Unfortunately, her mother died before the two could speak. Four months later, Josiane was operated on for a malignant tumor in her breast. She so badly wanted to hear a loving word from her mother! The breast is the organ that symbolizes symbiosis with or sometimes opposition to the mother. In both cases, the relationship lacks balance and fits into the "too much" or "not enough" category.

• A need for emotional security

Breast women have a hard time with emotional upheaval. They need stability and a secure, solid anchorage. In the wake of psycho-emotional trauma, some people show astonishing resilience. However, the breast woman is lost and doesn't know how to get herself back on track. She ends up finding solutions but often with great difficulty. This does not go without damage to her breasts, which retain the memory of the emotional stress and can develop tumors or other problems.

• Real or imagined loneliness

Even when they are not alone, some people experience an extreme feeling of loneliness. You can feel very much alone even if you have many friends and acquaintances. The problem is markedly more severe when the person lives alone. Their actual solitude reinforces this feeling of loneliness.

A patient who constantly developed cysts in her breasts told me one Monday, "You are the first person I've spoken to since Friday night. It's often like that on weekends. Sometimes I talk loudly to give the neighbors the impression that I have guests." This woman had moved to the city a few months earlier. Because she was shy and afraid to impose upon people, it was difficult for her to make friends.

• Breakups and difficult transitions

A partner leaving you, your children growing up and moving on, betrayal, any form of emotional blackmail, harassment at work—all are examples of breakups and emotions that can affect the breasts, the perfect target organ. The mere fear of being left or betrayed can create symptoms such as mastitis, cysts, inflammation, or cancer in the most severe cases. Certain families seem to cultivate this type of stress through constant confrontation, jealousy, and verbal violence, particularly between brothers and sisters. Badly negotiated "turns" in our life can occur in the intimate sphere, in the family, or in one's professional circle. Very often, women who live alone put everything into their job—it becomes their whole world. They put as much into it as they would into a family, so complications or insensitive reactions they may encounter at work seriously affect them.

Yvette led a peaceful life with her husband: few bumps, they got along great, and were considered a model couple by their friends. But one day her husband announced that he was leaving her for another woman he had loved for years, and who now was expecting a child with him. "It was as if lightning had struck me—the pain was indescribable, and the worst thing is that it was as if I already knew that something terrible was going to happen to me," Yvette says. Two years later, she had to have a mastectomy because of a tumor in her right breast. Again and again she asked me, "Do you think I made that tumor myself?"

It is important to understand that whether we are conscious of it or not, our emotions affect our organs. By educating oneself and applying the many ways to counterbalance the negative affects, one can increase the possibility for greater health.

• An unfulfilled wish to have a child

This can happen to women who are alone and have reached the critical age for child-bearing, or to mothers of several children who know that they won't have any more. The breast woman is acutely conscious of her age limitations for child-bearing. She knows it's too late but hangs on to an unreasonable hope. She doesn't want to get older. She would like to have more children. This sometimes manifests in the form of breast discharge, but much more frequently through breast congestion. The breasts seem to get larger, as if they were preparing to nurse.

• Feelings of guilt and failure

We build up guilt feelings on the basis of actual or imaginary facts. Here's another example from my practice: Marie was convinced that she had brought up her children poorly. Her in-laws fueled the feeling—they would criticize her for being "too permissive, too soft-hearted." Marie thought she had failed to give her children sufficient limits and barriers for them to become hard-working and disciplined pupils. A full-time mother, totally devoted to her children, she was ridden with feelings of guilt and failure and kept saying, "I should have…. I didn't do this, I forgot that, it's my fault…." Eventually she contracted breast cancer. It was caught in time, but she did require a mastectomy. After the operation, she decided to see a psychotherapist. Those guilt feelings are now "history" to her. And her in-laws no longer raise the subject of "how to raise the kids"!

Breast women can easily feel guilty for problems that are not their responsibility. Sandrine suddenly left her fiancé for no apparent reason. She found him "not enough of this and a bit too much of that." The years went by, and she remained alone. Around age forty-five, she began to feel despair at being single, constantly repeating that it was her fault: "I should have married that guy even if I wasn't totally convinced. My life is a desert, and only I am to blame." Never letting up on feeling guilty, Sandrine develops recurrent cysts in her breasts. She started therapy with a psychoanalyst. She is beginning to understand that deep down inside, she didn't want to live with a man. Her father was violent, and she thought that all men were like that. She would have almost found it normal for a man to beat her, and had often hit herself on the chest.

• Submission, fatalism

Breast women tend to be submissive—to their husband, their children, their parents, to a friend, a relative, an influential person…. Seeking perfection and the ideal relationship, they tend to submit to avoid clashes and to be accepted. Often rather fatalistic, they don't even question this attitude. "What can you do? That's the way it is!" you'll often hear them say.

• Difficulty finding their place

Breast people show a lack or a loss of reference points. Unlike lung people, who let other people enter or invade their territory, breast people don't know what territory to occupy. They go from one territory, position, or role to another, looking for their real place. Sometimes they do too much and sometimes not enough, asking questions like: "What kind of mother, wife, sister, doctor, waitress am I?" This lack of territoriality can also come from too strict an education as a child. They were told what to do and be. As an adult there is conflict between what they were told to be and what they feel like they want to be.

• Shyness

A woman's breasts are the most visible part of her thorax, exposed to everyone's sight and imagination. The development of breasts at puberty can be the source of problems in relating to others. There are cases of kyphosis (slouching, which can lead to hump back changes in the spine) that come from wanting to hide one's breasts: the teenage girl hunches her shoulders and back. When uncomfortable with her new femininity, she can be very shy in public. Her shyness can be coupled with aggression in certain situations. As we know, our childhood or teenage timidity can follow us for many years into adulthood. Often, it never leaves us.

• Wanting to look like an icon

We're talking about that unrealistic, idealized image that we see in cartoons or super-women magazines: a woman with silicone-filled breasts, entrancing and dominating. Nothing seems to resist her. She is an icon that symbolizes the power of femininity—the self-confident woman who pushes her chest (and large breasts) forward. Even if the breast woman doesn't totally identify with this type of image, she sometimes fantasizes about being this power-woman. There are now high-tech bras that make the breasts look larger and give perfect support. They help give a little boost to some women's self-confidence.

• Superficial serenity

Breast women put on a calm facade that reassures people around them. But things are not that simple: deep down inside, their need to be reassured is so strong that they project this feeling onto others. Jaqueline is a physical therapist, and her patients all say the same thing: "It's amazing how great a session with her makes me feel," "I go home confident in the future and ready to face anything." Jaqueline's general practitioner detects breast cancer during a routine checkup. "Why me? I've helped my patients so much. It's not fair...." By working with a psychoanalyst, she realizes that she actually did "too much" for other people, in part as a way of attempting to hide the insecurity deep inside herself. "I know, it's my mom and her mother who gave me that fear," she says in retrospect. "They were so strict, and were always warning me about the so-called dangers of life. I shouldn't have cheated and let everybody believe I was so calm," she recognizes.

Today Jaqueline is doing well. And her patients say she's changed: "If we're late she no longer gives us our session regardless of the time." She works less and goes on long trips. And most of all, Jaqueline has learned to make people respect her. She is no longer a victim of that obsessive need to make everybody happy and to be too nice.

How to Take Care of the Breasts

From a physical point of view

- The main thing is to see your general practitioner or your gynecologist regularly.
- Learn to self-examine your breasts, to locate painful or indurate (hardened) areas.
- Do not wear bras that are too tight.
- Do not hesitate to give your breasts a massage, in circular motions starting from below the breasts and going up the outer side.
- Exercise regularly. Practice stretching for your thorax and arms, because the breasts are organs that tend to get congested and to sag. They have no muscles of their own—they depend on the muscle tone of the chest for support. The breasts need to be carried by a chest that holds itself upright and is flexible. Stretching is recommended, as is working on your chest muscles with a light weight in each hand (a good exercise).

Exercise

- Standing, push your palms against each other. Count to 20, relax, and begin again.
- Work first with your hands close to your chest, then hold them further and further away to make the exercise more challenging.

From a nutritional point of view

- Eat fiber-rich vegetables and fruits: broccoli, string beans, peas, potatoes, endive, spinach, sorrel, leek, garlic, bananas, dates, coconut, raspberries, blackcurrants, watermelon, passion fruit, prunes. These foods can temper the production of estrogen, which in excess causes pain in the breasts. The same is true for all foods that contain a lot of omega-3 natural oils, such as flaxseeds, walnuts, salmon, and shrimp.
- Learn as much as you can (from both Western medicine and a naturopathic doctor) about birth control pills and hormone replacement therapy. When your liver is upset by excess estrogens which impede the proper excretion of the bile, it has trouble eliminating foods that naturally overburden it, such as chocolate, alcohol, cream, cold cuts, fried oils, and cheese. You may want to avoid these foods during ovulation and before your period if you have trouble with your breasts or other aspects of health.

French medical circles have long questioned the results of American and British statistics concerning the possible role of hormone replacement therapy in the development of breast cancer, yet even they are becoming more cautious and are applying the safety-first principle.

From a psychological point of view

Accept and show your femininity. A woman should feel beautiful to herself, in part due to what makes her physically different from men. The breasts and the pelvis are the manifest, visible elements of femininity. Some women complain of having small breasts and do everything they can to hide them; other women are embarrassed by their larger breasts and withdraw from the unwanted attention. Hunched back and shoulders and crossed arms are common protective attitudes.

Here's an analogy: The eyes are not beautiful simply because of their color—it's the whole effect, the way they glitter and shine. The same is true for a woman when she carries herself well and is proud of her femininity. If there is a serious psychological problem, one should see a therapist. This will be most beneficial if you also work on healing and/or enhancing your body through nutrition, exercise, and manual therapy as discussed in this book.

9

The Gallbladder:
A Small Pocketful of Annoyance

L ocated on the undersurface of the liver, the gallbladder is pear-shaped, roughly four inches long and one and one-half inches wide. The part that emerges beneath the liver is about the size of the end of your thumb. It is connected to the rest of the digestive system by a network of tubes that transport the bile, a greenish liquid, secreted by the liver.

How the Gallbladder Works

• It stores and concentrates bile

The liver produces one quart of bile a day, which is stored in the gall bladder. The gall bladder absorbs water from the bile and reduces it 10 – 20 % of original volume. It becomes a super-concentrate that the body can use according to need. The bile plays an essential role in digesting fats and eliminating cholesterol. It goes into action when our sight and smell are stimulated by food, and when our stomach dilates to receive food and drink. Upon this stimulus, the bile passes from the gall bladder into the duodenum via the cystic and the common bile ducts.

The bile, made up of residue produced by the liver, is brownish-green. You can see it when you "spit up bile." If the problem comes from the liver, the color is straw yellow. When you vomit, it's often the case that the gallbladder and the liver were disturbed by the products you swallowed or by your stress.

• It's a good stonemason

A gallstone is like a little pebble that forms in the gallbladder. Most of the time it is the result of cholesterol crystallizing when we have too much of it or when our bile salt level is too low. We can have gallstones and not even notice it. They don't cause any symptoms when they stay in the gallbladder. We feel pain only when the stones leave the gallbladder and migrate toward the bile ducts. When they get stuck inside the cystic canal (the gallbladder's first ejection route), the gallbladder can develop an inflammation. Occasionally gallstones may block the bile duct at the entrance to the duodenum, causing inflammation of the pancreas, which is adjacent.

Sometimes gallstone attacks can trigger pain in the most unexpected parts of the body, such as the ovaries or the appendix. Especially in women, estrogens (again!) make the bile thicker and more viscous, and therefore harder to eliminate.

When the Gallbladder Doesn't Work as well as It Should

You may notice:

- A heaviness or a stitch under the ribs on the right side. There can also be a sensitive area under the right shoulder blade.
- Cervical pain that starts up mainly on the left side, and then spreads to the entire neck.
- Hypersensitivity of smell and sight. The photosensitivity makes you want to wear dark glasses or hide from the light as soon as the sun comes out.
- Nausea, in some cases leading to vomiting (which frees the bile).
- Feeling repelled by fatty or strong-smelling foods.
- Trouble digesting, felt half an hour or an hour after meals.
- A vague smell of apple or acetone in the breath.

- Headaches that appear in anarchical attacks, often on weekends, when the pressure lets down.
- Mucous membrane problems, sinus infections, skin allergies, pimples, greasy hair.
- Irritability is a frequent reaction to a malfunctioning gallbladder.

~Gallbladder People~

Certain emotions or attitudes irritate the gallbladder. And conversely, an imbalance in the gallbladder has negative effects on our thoughts and attitudes. What is responsible, the emotion or the organ? If we take the time to reflect upon our actions and our lives, we can get to the bottom of it.

• Constant preoccupation

The gallbladder person is a worrier, but he or she usually worries about unimportant matters. There is always some little detail that isn't quite right or is likely to not be executed properly: "Did my son wake up on time? Will I be on time? Did I close the door properly? Where did I put my keys? Did I answer that letter?" To live in such a constant state of preoccupation can cause spasms or irritation in the gallbladder. Understandably, when the gallbladder is the weak link, the gallbladder person is even more anxious and worried.

• Mainly material stress

The gallbladder does not react to metaphysical preoccupations. The future of mankind and related anxiety are not its problem. It is affected by everyday, routine matters and mundane details.

• Annoyance

"The slightest little thing can irritate me," says the gallbladder person. When this becomes a chronic attitude, it almost always causes social and personal problems. Sylvie is on a ski trip with her husband. Trouble begins: "I don't know if I still fit into my ski outfit. My shoes hurt me last year—I'll surely have the same problem this year!" Sylvie gets restless. She can't face all these preoccupations. Her husband is ready and steps out of the chalet saying that he'll wait for her at the bottom of the ski run. She is annoyed but doesn't say anything. Five minutes later, she's finally ready, but she is missing her skis. "Where is my key to the ski locker? I have to call Jean. Oh no, my cell phone has run out of power!" Everything at once! A series of little details that keep kindling Sylvie's anxiety and ends up spoiling what should have been a pleasurable day. A person with the gallbladder as a weak link will become annoyed more easily than a person who does not have this imbalance. The emotion of annoyance irritates the gallbladder. And conversely, an imbalance in the gallbladder increases one's feeling of annoyance. As with all the organs and emotions, which came first, the chicken or the egg? That is the question, and the reason to learn about these amazing connections. By carefully looking at one's lifestyle and situation, you can solve that puzzle. At the same time, by working on one or the other (the organ or the emotion), you can reverse the self-perpetuating loop that can be created when dis-ease is present.

• Hypersensitivity and hyperactivity

Gallbladder people have "raw nerves." The slightest remark vexes them. Show them a spot on their coat or mention an equivocal attitude on their part, and you might set off a drama. When I work with such people, I have to watch my words because they can be easily misinterpreted. For instance, when I asked a patient "Have you had oily skin for a long time?" she answered, offended, "What? Oily skin? I wash all the time!"

• Fear of conflict, even minor

Seeing two people argue is enough to trouble a gallbladder person. They seem to be very sensitive to atmospheres and to the negative energy that certain situations can produce. That is the case with Florence. She does water aerobics (a highly recommended form of exercise) with a trainer who has a bad temper: whenever the water isn't warm enough, someone arrives late for the class, people don't do the movements properly, or she catches people talking, the instructor blows up. The stress physically affects Florence's gallbladder, and she would frequently feel a painful spot under her ribs, on the right side, when she left her water aerobics class in a bad mood. Finally Florence switched to another pool, with another trainer. She feels much better. Life is complicated enough as it is—why add on unnecessary stress?

• A need to stay in one place

Even if they are attracted by travel, gallbladder people don't like to change their habits. They need their "little world" and their usual references around them. Having everything in its place reassures them. A trip coming up? Panic! They accumulate stress over the most minute practical details. They are afraid of being late, or of having forgotten something. They are afraid of planes. They can become pale or drenched in sweat when the plane takes off or lands. It isn't unusual for them to have an upset stomach after the trip.

• Departures and separations are very hard to accept

When going away becomes an ordeal, the gallbladder is the first organ to react (for most people, but more intensely for gallbladder people). It's the same thing with difficult separations. The person feels a small tense lump beneath the liver. However, in the case of really painful, not to speak of heartbreaking, departures and separations, the heart takes over and can really suffer.

• Fear of exams and confrontation

For gallbladder people, any test is a source of great anxiety and extraordinary stress. Luc has to take his driving test tomorrow. He is stressed out beyond all proportion. An attack of reactive diarrhea "wrenches his bowels." He feels weak, has no confidence in his knowledge, and thinks that he won't remember a thing. He is creating additional pressure on himself. And even if, deep down inside, Luc thinks he will pass the test, he tells everyone that he's going to fail. The tension rises to a peak until the fatal moment—the test. Suddenly he calms down, and he passes the test! "All that stress for nothing! I'll never learn," Luc finally confesses.

> ### • *Extreme punctuality*

Gallbladder people are almost obsessively punctual. They can't stand being late, or other people being late.

> ### • *Slightly jealous*

Extreme ups and downs (a "manic-depressive" tendency) can characterize a gallbladder person, and they sometimes bear grudges. They act jealous when they don't feel equal to another person, perhaps a rival! People with a sensitive gallbladder prefer stable and peaceful relationships, but sometimes they are the ones who provoke conflict!

How to Take Care of the Gallbladder

From a physical point of view

- Get into the habit of doing breathing exercises. Try stretching, which is an excellent way of relaxing the body and the gallbladder. If necessary, see a relaxation therapist, who will help you strengthen your defenses in regard to stress.
- Learn how to give yourself a massage under the right-side ribs. Start from the navel and go up toward your ribs until you feel a sensitive, perhaps even very sensitive, area. Stay in that area, doing very light circular movements. When the massage is done properly and in the right place, it will make you produce saliva—a conditional reflex.
- Consider seeing a practitioner of Visceral Manipulation. He or she can influence the gallbladder. Feeling with their fingers delicately under the thorax, a therapist can relax the tensions in the wall of the gallbladder when it goes through spasms in a tense and oversensitive state. He or she can also "drain" the gallbladder, to encourage eliminating bile and tiny gallstones. At the beginning of the session, the gallbladder will react very strongly, and

then, little by little, it relaxes and the patient feels relief. The next day the patient may feel a slight tiredness and a sensitivity in the liver area. In any case, this manual therapy is an excellent technique, recommended for anyone, not just gallbladder people.

From a nutritional point of view

The foods to be avoided are the same as for the liver (as you'll see in the next chapter):

- Chocolate. It's hard to determine what exactly is the harmful ingredient that goes into its making, but one thing is certain: it is no friend of the liver or the gallbladder.
- Cooked cream. You can replace it with milk, soy, or rice cream.
- Sulfur-based preservatives. They are indicated on certain packages and are commonly called sulfites. (See the advice and recommendations in Chapter 10 below, on the liver, page 111.) Careful—wines contain sulfites, but due to a special waiver, producers are not obliged to indicate it. Certain foods have no added sulfites but are sprayed with them for better preservation. This is the case with peanuts, almonds, and other appetizer nuts.

From a psychological point of view

Since annoyances cause blockage in the gallbladder, do everything to avoid them. Easy to say, but how? Here are a few examples:

- Take a little more time to prepare and to get wherever you're going, in order to spare yourself the rush and stress of being late.
- Carefully prepare for trips, moves, and changes in your life.

- Whenever possible, avoid staying in places where clashes are underway. At home, if an argument is going on in the kitchen, take refuge in the living room, or go out for a walk. Don't seek out tension, especially if you're not at your best and you already feel tense.

10

The Liver:
Our Deeper Self and Emotions

The liver is a major organ, both in size and because of its essential functions which enable survival. Moreover, it is one of the key organs in our emotional life. Its average weight of about 3.3 pounds makes it one of the heaviest organs in our body, slightly heavier than the brain. It is situated largely to the right, under the ribs and above the intestines. Usually the liver can be felt under the protective edge of the rib cage. A real chemical plant, the liver is (to put it humorously) our Poison Control Center. It filters out all toxic substances. Whenever we consume anything in excess, the liver separates the wheat from the chaff and transforms toxins into less harmful substances. But don't over-abuse its miraculous powers. The liver might end up playing tricks on you!

This organ also plays a major role in our biliary (bile-producing) and hormonal systems. It is one of the main regulators of digestive metabolism, and is an "energy reserve" organ, as the list below indicates.

- The liver stores iron, vitamin B12, and the folic acid that is so good for our hair.
- It takes part in balancing our glycemia by storing sugar and turning it into reserve fatty acids, which makes the sugar particularly useful.
- It metabolizes and balances protein and nitrogenous waste.
- It stores and metabolizes fats.

How the Liver Works

All the digestive organs work together. When one of them fails, the entire digestive system suffers. It's like an automobile assembly line: one faulty part is enough for a vehicle to come out defective at the end of the line. The liver's role is to neutralize toxic substances.

• The bile

In twenty-four hours, the liver produces close to a quart of bile that is partly concentrated and stocked by the gallbladder. The bile works as a detergent, emulsifying the fat content in our food. It segments fats into very fine droplets, so fine that they can easily blend with the water in the intestines. That is what emulsion is: small particles of one liquid in suspension in another liquid. Milk, for example, is an emulsion of fat in water. The bile is made up of water, cholesterol, and bile salts. The bile salts play a role in absorbing digested fats, cholesterol (HDL and LDL), and certain vitamins (A, D, E, and K). This task is performed together with the pancreas. The bile salts also deodorize the fecal matter; when feces or gases offend our sense of smell, it is a sign that the liver isn't functioning to the best of its abilities.

• The famed cholesterol

Contrary to general belief, you should know that three-quarters of our cholesterol is produced by the liver; the remaining quarter comes from foods of animal origin. We have to distinguish between the good and the bad kind when talking about this so-called "enemy" of the arteries. LDL (low-density lipoprotein) is the bad kind, the one that deposits onto the walls of the arteries and creates a risk of clogging them up. HDL (high-density lipoprotein) is the good kind that fights its "brother" by cleaning up the very same arteries. It's like the battle between David and Goliath! (See also page 115.)

• The hormones

The liver is one of the main factors in the formation of sexual hormones (estrogen, progesterone, testosterone). One of its tasks is to eliminate excess hormones, especially estrogens, which have a tendency to irritate the liver and make it overly sensitive.

• Vitamins, proteins, and carbohydrates

The liver produces and stocks a lot of vitamins and enzymes (the latter are responsible for making our digestive juices work efficiently). The blood that goes through the liver comes out enriched with enzymes, which make it possible to digest carbohydrates, to disintegrate albumin (protein), and to better assimilate fats and hormones. The pancreas helps the liver store, transform, and release carbohydrates in useable form for the body. The liver also transforms certain carbohydrates into triglycerides, that is to say, fats.

Thanks to the bile it secretes, the liver synthesizes proteins and breaks them down into elements which the body can more easily assimilate. Protein is indispensable to human survival, because it is needed in the formation and repair of cells. But the body is incapable of producing protein by itself. This is why the liver plays such a pivotal and foundational role. It makes use of whatever the body needs and transforms excess proteins into urea, which is then eliminated by the kidneys.

The liver also takes part in producing vitamin D, which is required to absorb calcium. It transforms carotene (a yellow or red pigment in vegetables such as carrots) into vitamin A. It regulates the iron content in the red blood cells, thereby helping to prevent anemia (a decrease of red blood cells).

• And that's not all ...

The liver has many other functions. It is simultaneously our minister of economy, of family affairs, of construction, and of health, and it takes part in every battle, on all fronts where excesses are involved, helping to eliminate them. When intoxicated by detrimental matter we have ingested or breathed in, the liver immediately becomes congested and sensitive. Do you know that when you paint a room, it's your liver that's in charge of ridding your body of all those toxic substances contained in paint fumes? And there are a lot of them! This is why painters sometimes develop liver disease. (If you need to paint or apply varnish, put on a mask and air the room as much as possible.) When you have an infection, it is the liver that takes care of ridding you of all viruses, germs, and other undesirable boarders. Any disturbance will curb its normal functions, and immediate signs of fatigue will appear.

• *The liver in women*

Marie-Claude comes to me for a pain in her right shoulder. "It's strange," she says, "I didn't fall. It just started suddenly one morning, for no reason. I saw a doctor who diagnosed periarthritis of the shoulder."

"What treatment did he prescribe?" I asked, with little doubt as to what the answer would be.

"Pain-killers and anti-inflammation medicine which give me stomach pains and makes me nauseous," Marie-Claude answers.

I notice that her complexion is slightly yellow, her hair a bit oily and flat, her skin shiny. Palpation reveals a sensitivity in the liver and gallbladder area. My hand is not attracted toward her shoulder, but toward her liver: "It must be the liver," I surmise.

"How could the liver give me a shoulder ache?!" she exclaims, doubtfully.

"Simply because it is linked to your shoulder via its nervous system. Tell me: in the morning when you wake up, do you feel OK? Does the daylight hurt your eyes? Are you hungry? Is your hair oilier than usual? You are fifty-one—is your period still regular?"

While answering my questions, Marie-Claude begins to realize that her liver actually is having a hard time doing its job. I explain a bit more: "One of the liver's tasks is to eliminate estrogen. Since your period is not regular, it looks like you are going through some hormone imbalance between progesterone and estrogen. So it's absolutely normal for your liver to be reacting. It is actually intoxicated and can no longer eliminate the food you eat properly, especially since you say that you're a chocolate addict. Your liver is begging for mercy! It's letting you know. It's congested, and it is irritating your sensory nervous system that transmits pain to your shoulder via a network of nerve fibers which connects the two."

Without even touching her shoulder, I work on the liver, below the ribs on the right side, and compress and decompress the gallbladder area to drain it. Her shoulder begins to regain some amplitude of movement. "But be careful," I warn. "No more chocolate, cream, or doughnuts, and don't go near alcohol. Eat as many fruits and vegetables as possible. Drink water often and a little at a time. Walk regularly, and come back to see me in a month." The next time she comes, Marie-Claude assures me that she has followed my advice. Indeed, the pain has disappeared and her shoulder has regained its mobility.

This is not an isolated case. In our practice we see a lot of shoulder periarthritis in women in their early fifties, because estrogen peaks literally poison the liver. Men also can develop periarthritis as a symptom of liver irritation. However, menopause especially pre-disposes women to this problem.

• Relays throughout the body

Nervous circuits sometimes follow what seem to be strange routes in the human body. For instance, the liver is linked to the elbow. Tendonitis and tennis elbow can actually come from a liver problem.

Jean-Paul loves to do little jobs around the house. Drills and screwdrivers, pliers and hammers hold no secrets for him. But one day he notices a persistent pain in his right elbow. After trying all the usual creams and pills in vain, he comes to me. His elbow is slightly swollen and hurts when I touch it. He also has a cervical stiffness on the same (right) side. Part of the liver's nervous centers actually begin at the lower cervical vertebrae. I explain to this patient that the elbow is a relay between the cervical spine and the liver, because both of them have nerves ending in the elbow. Therefore, I can help his elbow by reducing his cervical tension. I add that it's important for me to know what he eats, because the liver can send on its own discomfort to the elbow. Jean-Paul says that he drinks no alcohol, doesn't eat too many sweet foods, but he confesses that he's a big cheese eater, and that he prefers cheese to any other food, especially at supper. "Try to stop eating cheese in the evening," I suggest. "Within a few weeks you'll be able to use your elbow painlessly again."

In Jean-Paul's case, this small change was enough to break the vicious cycle of elbow-cervical-liver-elbow-cervical. By treating his cervical tension and changing his diet, Jean-Paul found that his liver could get better. We all have arthritis to some degree, due to the aging of our cartilage and/or the consequences of trauma. In addition poor eating habits, which make the liver and kidneys overwork can promote arthritis. In the case of this patient, acting on different aspects of the problem at the same time allowed his body to eliminate and to clean itself up a little. When our liver works better, life looks brighter!

Why Take Care of Your Liver?

As with all parts of our body, we owe the liver attention and care. A healthy liver is a guarantee of buoyant physical and intellectual activity and a resilient state of mind. What is better than a good dose of *joie de vivre* to carry on your life with a positive attitude, to undertake things with enthusiasm and to the best of your capacities? When you feel good in your body, you feel good in your head! Sure of your values and your personality, you'll be able to assert them and to make clear choices. An engorged or intoxicated liver tires the body more than usual. You immediately feel exhausted; you can just barely keep up your everyday activities, with minimal energy, and more than that seems impossible to you. Remember how you feel the day after a party where you drank a lot of alcohol—not too great, right? So imagine that same feeling, every day, because of poor eating habits. It could indicate that you are not paying enough attention and respect to yourself, and you are harming your health and personality.

When poorly treated, the liver lets you know

One of my patients, a writer, had just finished a novel—a year's worth of regular and persistent labor. When he re-read the whole manuscript, he noticed a lack of cohesion in certain chapters that fell short of the flow of the rest of the book. Intrigued by this breach in coherence, he tried to remember when he had written the incriminating chapters. He recalled that he had worked on them during holidays at friends' homes, where he had eaten and drunk (alcohol) more than usual.

When the Liver Isn't Working as well as It Should

Among the warning symptoms of a liver problem, you'll recognize a few, because they'll seem so familiar. Others are more subtle, and even if you feel them, you may not be able to associate them with a particular organ.

• Headaches

Liver problems can result in either migraine headaches in one half of the face and head, or general headaches affecting the entire head. Migraines often come with other discomforts: a nauseous feeling, a need to hide from light and noise, feeling worn out, etc.

• Eyesight problems

When you wake up, the light is hard to bear. This photophobia is caused by dysfunction of the liver and can even lead to a slight loss of your visual acuity. On some days, it may be difficult to read small print.

• Oily hair and dandruff

Your hair gets oily. Dandruff appears. You have to wash your hair frequently. This is often an indicator of poor liver function.

• Hypersensitive skin

Skin is sensitive to the point of becoming allergic. Soaps, shampoos, and dishwashing detergents that never used to cause you any problem suddenly set off skin reactions. Even if you don't have acne, pimples and red patches appear on your face.

• A white and coated tongue

Upon arising in the morning, one's tongue can be seen to have a white coat of mucus on its surface.

• Bad breath

The odor seems "heavy," as if lingering traces of what you ate yesterday were coming out of your mouth.

• Perspiration

Perspiration (sweating) is more abundant, appears with the slightest effort, and has a strong, unpleasant smell.

• A hypersensitive sense of smell

One's ability to smell things becomes oversensitive. We turn into a hunting dog, with a very developed flair! Unpleasant smells disgust us. Even certain very fine perfumes can make us nauseous.

• Sensitive gums

The areas around the teeth become oversensitive and reactive, bleeding easily. They may even become infected.

• Irritated mucous membranes

Irritated and congested mucous membranes can lead to sinus infections and bronchial congestion, both of which can indicate a dysfunctional liver. Congested mucous membranes can cause snoring. Did you know that consuming alcohol or chocolate can cause a sinus infection in certain people, the very next day or two days later, as well as a morning cough?

• Dark-colored urine

It is the color of very strong tea.

• A dull, muddy complexion

When the liver is out of balance, this will show up on the person's complexion.

• Physical fatigue

When the liver is overburdened, we're not in brilliant shape, to say the least. The slightest effort costs us a lot of energy and makes us sweat profusely.

Athletes don't perform as well

Athletes don't perform as well with compromised liver function, and their best results get scarcer, despite intense training. If they watch their diet, they can regain those tenths of a point (or whatever margin) and restore their resistance. Just one glass of alcohol the night before a race can make a skier or a sprinter lose precious hundredths of a second.

• Insomnia

Sleep is interrupted by several wake phases. Dreams turn into nightmares. Some people dream of being pursued by dangerous maniacs, and their legs refuse to carry them when they try to run away. When it is overworked, the liver heats up, and you might feel it between midnight and two o'clock in the morning.

• Sleep that brings no rest

With a poorly treated liver, don't count on recharging your batteries during the night! Waking up becomes very difficult, and you feel emptied out.

• Vertigo

Often vertigo has nothing to do with the inner ear but comes from the liver. Feeling dizzy, unstable, as if wrapped in cotton, can be linked to the liver. Some specialists also speak of an inflammation in the mucous membranes inside the inner ear, and of stasis of the veins, which slightly diminishes the volume of blood circulating in the veins.

• Difficult digestion

You start by saying, "I didn't digest that too well," and then, if the discomfort persists, "I have a poor stomach, I don't digest well." In fact, digestion requires a lot of energy. And you are lacking resources! You feel a heaviness on the right side. After a meal, it is hard for you to keep your eyes open. If you're home, and you sit down in an armchair or lie down on the couch, you'll definitely fall asleep.

• Intellectual fatigue

Don't go for any transcendent thoughts when your liver isn't functioning well! Just take care of daily matters. The liver looks for energy wherever it can find it, especially in the brain. Your intellectual capacity will suffer.

• A decrease in fighting spirit

That combative spirit which makes champions and winners is lacking when the liver doesn't work well. This is crucial for people committed to excellence, such as high-level athletes. It's no easier for the rest of us, and just as crucial, when we have to make the right decisions at the right moment.

At this level of ill health, if we don't become aware of the state we are in and don't regain the upper hand, physical—and in resonance with it, psychological—dis-ease will settle in. Various disagreeable symptoms result from poor liver function such as the ones listed above as well as more serious troubles: allergies, sinus problems, pyorrhea, loosening of the teeth, hemorrhoids, muscular problems (straining, tendonitis) due to insufficient elimination of lactic acid, pain in the joints (especially the right shoulder), frequent sprains due to a lack of attentiveness, poor job performance, and depression. If one or several of these symptoms persist, it is time to act to improve your well-being and health on a long-term basis.

~Liver People~

Depending on genes and especially on poor eating habits, the liver sets off specific attitudes and emotional reactions. Of course, no single person has all the signs at once. When signs are present, it is to a varying degree. The liver is the main organ representing our inner being and "I" self.

The mind and the liver

Sometimes our mind is so deeply troubled that it sends its pain on to an organ, usually to our weak link. The liver is the receptor of family guilt and the concerns of our deeper self. This is obvious in numerous cases, among them Geneviève, a woman who is very dependent upon her mother. She never makes a decision without consulting her—an inescapable mother, a parent but also a mentor and a judge who, unfortunately, dies suddenly. A few months after her death, Geneviève suffers from liver symptoms. Tests confirm that her liver is in trouble: it is congested and has difficulty purifying and eliminating waste. Medicine, diet, nothing seems to help. Discouraged, she finally ends up at my practice, hoping that Visceral Manipulation treatment of her liver will alleviate her troubles. The treatment doesn't bring sufficient improvement. In our profession, we have to measure our limits quickly. It is best not to be stubborn and to find another solution for the patient. After questioning her at length, I advised her to see a psychotherapist, which she did. Psychotherapy was the right remedy. Geneviève needed help to stop feeling guilty: she felt that not enough had been done to help save her mother. Her psyche had gotten the better of her liver.

According to his or her genetic code and life story, every individual has a personal, intrinsic value. We build up our personalities alone, without any makeup or artifice. It is our deeper self that evaluates, thinks, decides, and makes plans without trying to position itself in relation to others—with its good qualities and its faults, of course, but without any theatrics or ostentation. Some people try to put off this meeting with themselves as long as possible, or they always act according to pre-established and approved social codes. When a teenager rebels, it's precisely because he or she is trying to assert his or her personality and to exist in relation to others.

Most people just follow the tracks: it's simple—the locomotive leads us to our destination. It is more difficult to follow our own track, the one our personality reveals to us. This approach demands real investment. The inner self is often opposed to appearances. Nevertheless, appearances are useful; we all have a social role to fulfill. Whether we are the chairman of a company, a doctor, a nurse, a shopkeeper, a civil servant, or a teacher, we all follow the rules of our profession. Contrary to the old saying, "It is not the cowl that makes the monk," the same person, depending on whether they are wearing a worker's overalls or a suit and tie, will have a different appearance, gait, and authority. Clothes give an appearance that can be very different from one's true nature. Our social activity shapes us. But the inner self can put on worker's overalls or a suit and tie without losing its identity. The problem arises when our social appearance unconsciously stifles our inner self.

We all meet with our inner self at some point, usually not before adulthood. Those who don't ever get that far may lack courage, or perhaps they simply don't feel the need. One of my patients, a brilliant businessman, comes for a routine checkup once a year. Ritually, I ask him, "What's new?" With jubilation and a great wealth of details, he describes his new car to me. To each his life: it doesn't keep him from being a nice guy!

• A hard time knowing oneself

Most people who have been through a dramatic event—the death of a loved one, a breakup, or a natural catastrophe—undergo a fundamental change in their view of life. They think differently and acquire an acute sense of the relativity of people and things. Sometimes the dramatic event precipitates this meeting with one's inner self. "Don't take life too seriously, you won't come out alive anyway!" Pretty black humor, but this phrase does convey a sure sense of derision. Yet the way our personality, attitudes, and thoughts develop should be taken seriously. Dysfunction of the liver doesn't bar all roads to self-knowledge. Things are more subtle. The meeting with oneself can occur, but not in a continuous and harmonious way when the liver is not working as well as it should. Deep personal growth will be more painful, and will happen in stages.

• Dependency on the mother and on the past

Theoretically, we're all more or less dependent on our mother. It becomes less symbiotic when we grow up. But too great an attachment, not to mention subjection, will impair our own development. You can't say, "It's because my liver doesn't work well that I am too dependent on my mother." But dysfunction of the liver does cause doubt and uncertainty concerning the future and makes us lean toward the past. It is less frightening to look back without raising any questions than to project into an uncertain future, which would require commitment and responsibility. When we constantly delve into the past, we usually end up finding fault with our mother: she is a favored target of our past because of the central role she played. Paradoxically, it's often the case that the stronger the recriminations, the more intense the attachment and love.

One of my patients, Françoise, has an addictive need to call her mother. "The conversation always begins pleasantly," she tells me. "But inevitably, something will make me broach a touchy subject—like I know we don't agree on education, but I'll raise the subject anyway. Although the conversation gets pretty heated, I can't help being finicky, until my mother becomes exasperated and hangs up. I sometimes get the impression that she acts exactly the same way. But we do love each other!" Françoise admits that when she is feeling well, her latent aggressiveness stays put, and her phone calls with her mother are warmer. Françoise suffered from hepatitis A, a liver disease, which she caught on a trip abroad.

• Bad memories

The liver memorizes every element that goes into building our identity: emotions, pitfalls, death of loved ones, misadventures, illnesses, little joys, major happy events, and so on. From our birth until the moment we are going through now, the liver is one of the top organ witnesses to our most important emotions and life's course. When there is liver dysfunction, the bad memories very often come back and weaken us. They tarnish our actions and darken the road we still have left to travel. Negative elements and failures from our past do not give us the confidence we need to dare face similar situations in the future. We're afraid to repeat them. It's only human.

• A tendency toward pessimism, fear of the future

We've all experienced this: the day after a heavy meal, we don't usually feel very cheerful. We tend to see the dark side of things. If you keep on eating everything your liver dislikes, you will be overwhelmed with negative ideas and become the perfect example of the eternal pessimist. In that frame of mind, how could you feel confident about the future? These bouts of pessimism start out being sporadic, but then they settle in, to the point of affecting the people around you and making them unhappy.

Popular belief has it that there are two kinds of doctors: the "great!" doctors, who say that everything is fine, and "terrible!" doctors, who only see what's wrong. Let's bet that the second kind has a liver problem.

• Lack of self-esteem

A dysfunctional liver can affect one's self-esteem, which is the ground we build ourselves on. We have to love ourselves to be able to love others well. Various circumstances can harm self-esteem: the relationship with parents and/or partner, one's place in the hierarchy at work, one's physical attributes or more superficial signals of fashion, etc. Some people have the type of personality that affects us negatively by gradually making us feel inadequate. Self-doubt and lack of self-esteem inhibit us greatly. Sometimes we'll react the opposite way: we'll try to force events or relationships, getting into power trips whereby the means justifies the end, which will supposedly compensate for our lack of self-esteem.

• A prisoner of routine

Few events in life offer us a chance to surpass ourselves, to be the movie hero who saves humankind. But we can surpass ourselves regularly at a more modest level—for example, by leaving the tracks we comfortably set our lives on, and taking some risks to change our habits. Deep inside, something guides us. We listen or don't listen to that little voice encouraging us to go beyond our usual routine, to transcend our ruts. It can mean going on an initiatory journey to get away from our usual pattern and try to regain our life force. We can also take up a humanitarian cause, simply helping people who need it, without boasting or bravado.

• Bad moods and ill-being

Guy comes to my practice one morning, tense and worn out, short of breath: "There, you have it," he says abruptly. "I have a pain in my neck that goes straight down into my shoulder, elbow, and fingers. I must have pulled a muscle last night in bed." He embarks upon a rather confused monologue: "I'm not doing well. First of all, it hurts. Plus, I had an argument with my wife over nothing. I'm always the one who takes out the dog. Actually, I wonder if it wasn't the dog who hurt me by pulling on the leash. My wife often makes these hurtful remarks, like 'You should take better care of the way you look' and 'You're no Brad Pitt, you know.' At work, I get the feeling they think I'm inefficient. Generally speaking, my life is no piece of cake...."

I take a look at his body as a whole. (It's important that a bodyworker not focus exclusively on the symptoms.) With Guy, the simple act of getting undressed and lying down causes a release of strong-smelling sweat. Of course his neck, muscles, and nerves, from the cervical area down into the arm, are very sensitive, even painful. Irresistibly my hand is attracted to the liver area: it is tense, congested, and hypersensitive. I tell him, "You definitely have a problem in your joints, linked to arthritis and neuralgia in the cervical and arm area [irritation of the nerves that go from the neck to the arm]. This is all reinforced by an overburdened liver. You should go for a complete medical checkup, and focus on what you can do on your own for your liver."

"That's true," Guy mused. "I eat too much fat, too much cheese, too much sugar, and a little glass here and there helps me cheer up."

For someone to admit an alcohol addiction is not easy. If they haven't yet admitted it or remain touchy about it, you have to approach the subject with care and kindness. I told Guy as I began to work on him: "I am going to ease your pain by carefully relaxing your muscles, nerves, and joints. But you can help yourself best. For one month, watch your diet. Try to eat more healthily, and to resist alcohol in any form. Eat as many fruits and vegetables as possible. Drink water often and in small quantities. Walk, and come back to see me. You have to hold out four weeks."

A month later, he's back, with a twinkle in his eye and standing straight. "You know what? I made it," Guy says, rather proudly. "My wife and I talked a lot, and she helped me. Less sauce, less fat. We went on the diet together. At work, people told me that I seemed more present. That made me happy."

"And what about your aches and pains?" I query.

"Better, much better. I feel well. But the hardest thing is the alcohol."

I gave Guy the address of a relaxation therapist who could help him face his addiction. The consultation was beneficial to him. This patient had chosen the right moment. He needed to hear the truth he couldn't face by himself.

This example shows some of the possible consequences of a poorly functioning liver: loss of ambition and creativity, not feeling good about oneself generally or when in the company of other people, self-deprecation, and physical pain. An unhealthy liver doesn't make us the best companion or partner. Everything becomes a problem, and we tend to provoke tensions and conflicts.

• Lack of a fighting spirit

Words like "combatant" and "fighter" generally make us think of someone who overcomes opponents through sheer force. But there is such a thing as "peaceful combat," where the "fight" is about our own capacity to surpass ourselves. For example, André is eighty-two and loves to go skiing whatever the weather. Hard snow or obstacles to jump over don't intimidate him. And this worries his family terribly. But he won't listen to them. Says André, "I don't do it to annoy them. It's for myself, to feel and test my strength."

Winter comes around, and André catches viral hepatitis from seafood. He gets over it with difficulty, and confides, "True, I'm tired, but it's mainly in my mind that things aren't going well. The proof is, I've resigned, I won't go skiing anymore. I don't want to take risks anymore."

• Absence of or decrease in creativity

Everybody is creative, to a certain degree. The architect who designs an innovative and ambitious project, the maid who irons shirts quicker and better than anyone else, the philosopher who writes a pamphlet against a certain school of thought—everyone is important in their field.

To be creative, our organism needs to be in optimal balance. People with a congested liver can manage their everyday life, but they tend to lack the energy to surpass themselves in any kind of creative endeavor. You might object that certain poets, painters, or musicians revealed their genius under the influence of alcohol (very toxic for the liver). They did so at a point where their body still had enough resources to compensate for it. But they often had hard lives, and many legendary substance-abusing artistic types ended their lives in difficulty and too soon. You might think of Verlaine, Rimbaud, Utrillo, and closer to our times, Serge Gainsbourg, a great twentieth-century songwriter. During an interview he complained about the ills of alcohol, which had "eaten up his composing abilities." He even concluded by saying, "The main thing is: don't drink!" Many of us regret that these artists didn't live longer, to go on delighting us with their talent.

• A feeling of insecurity

As we've already said, there are different degrees of fear. The most intense fears affect our kidneys, whereas feelings of insecurity (not so much actual danger) strongly influence the liver. Insecurity can cause paroxysmal attacks (sharp spasms) that only exacerbate the natural pessimism of people with a sensitive liver.

Marie-Claude's husband is a traveling salesman. Whenever he goes on a trip, she is overwhelmed with trepidation that something might happen to him. She is my patient and tells me, "When I'm not feeling well, it gets really bad. I have to bear with it and convince myself not to call him every half-hour. When I'm feeling OK, I don't have as hard a time with his being away." Then one day her husband had a car accident, and she exclaimed, "I felt it!" But she was forgetting that this feeling was with her constantly: that day, just as every other day, she had foreseen an accident. Marie-Claude suffers from a hormonal imbalance. Her body produces too many estrogens which her liver has trouble eliminating. This is not to say that her anxiety is due only to her liver problems: general oversensitivity and a difficult life are obvious contributors. But it is amplified by her liver dysfunction.

• Greater susceptibility

Watch your words with liver people when they aren't in good shape. They blow up over nothing. The slightest remark can trigger a huge fit of anger. It is never out of meanness. But the insecurity, fear, lack of confidence, and pessimism that are typical of liver dysfunction make the person hypersensitive. Choose the right moment to make a joke, because it might turn against you!

• Fits of anger

Angry outbursts are cyclical and practically inevitable. Strangely enough, once the person has expressed this anger, he or she feels better. We could compare this anger to a safety valve. The anger lets accumulated tensions loose, like a steam valve on a pressure cooker. There's nothing worse than "swallowed" and repressed anger that turns to rancor.

My patient Pierre comes to mind. He is a charming man, valued by his colleagues. He sometimes seems touchy, but it blows over quickly. Helpful, amiable, he usually has a good word for everyone. But his wife doesn't see things quite like that. Says she, "It's true he's nice, but sometimes I don't recognize him. He gets furious over details. When he comes home from work, most of the time he barely speaks—maybe just a few grunts in answer to my questions."

The liver is Pierre's weak link. When our liver isn't working the way it should, we generally feel tense and aggressive, and this is the case with Pierre. Even if he values his wife, he has a hard time tolerating her when his liver problems flare up.

• Little phobias

Some liver people have bouts of phobic behavior that can go from claustrophobia (fear of crowds and/or small, closed spaces) to agoraphobia (fear of open spaces). As a typical example, they might feel very uncomfortable in supermarkets. Of course, the tendency is within the person, but liver dysfunction cycles will prompt and reinforce it.

• Depression

The liver and the brain like to exchange their energies. When one of them is lacking energy, it takes it from the other. A bad liver pretty much means feeling blue! Liver dysfunction doesn't entail real depression, but it gives people a feeling of being drained, unhappy, unloved, inadequate, and lacking drive.

How to Take Care of the Liver

From a physical point of view

- Turkish baths and saunas are highly recommended—not to lose weight (it doesn't work) but to help eliminate toxins via the urine and sweat. Turkish baths (steam baths) have the advantage of making you lose very little water, because the body absorbs the surrounding humidity through breathing.
- Be knowledgeable and cautious about the medications you ingest, especially if you are a liver person. Many medicines are toxic for the liver. If you have a sensitive liver, you must tell your doctor (who should ask) when he prescribes drugs such as Tylenol, anti-depressants, and anti-anxiety medicine. All medicines are metabolized by the liver and kidneys and can be a cause of organ

dysfunction, sometimes serious (such as hepatitis). Birth control pills and hormone replacement therapy are definite risk factors. The liver becomes exhausted from having to eliminate the excess hormones and can no longer properly digest heavy foods; this leads to digestive problems, anxiety, and depression.

From a nutritional point of view

Certain foods are good for your liver (see list below), and your eating habits are a relatively easy avenue for change. Be particularly careful if you are overweight.

- *Chew:* The simple act of slowly chewing carbohydrates and protein helps us digest them and is less taxing for the body.
- You know it, and your body may have already shouted it to you—refrain from or enjoy moderately: French fries, doughnuts, and all other fried foods! Be sparing with cheese, fatty meats, pastry, chocolate, and cream (cooked). And of course, don't overdo alcohol.
- If you regularly drink more than a glass of alcohol per meal, your liver might end up playing tricks on you, sooner or later.
- Say yes to water. It is important to drink adequate water, preferably lukewarm. You can add a couple of drops of lemon to the water (three or four per glass) or drink green tea. Don't force yourself to drink two or three quarts of water, as some people recommend. The amount of water your body needs depends on your weight, height, sex, level of physical activity, and the season. Drink often and in small sips, more when you are active (such as hiking, working hard, and playing sports) or after a big meal if you consume lots of wine. Dark, strong-smelling urine is an indicator that you are not drinking and eliminating sufficient water. It's good to keep a bottle of water handy.

- Watch out for sulfites, common sulfur-based preservatives
in food and drink that can cause headaches and sinus
irritations. Wine producers have a special exemption
from European rules; they don't mention the presence
of sulfites in their ingredients. So observe how your
liver reacts to certain wines, champagnes, beers, and
fruit juices. Raw white cabbage or peeled potatoes
sold in supermarkets, salted and whitened cod, certain
frozen products (check the labels), mustard, vinegar, and
mayonnaise all contain sulfites that can stress your liver.
Some signs of liver overload include headaches, irritability,
fatigue, nausea, digestive disturbances (bloating,
constipation), inflammation, irritated and watery eyes,
hypertension, PMS and other hormonal imbalances, as
well as skin break-outs.

I remember one of my patients, who was very keen on natural prod-ucts, coming into my office with a package of apricots. "Look how beau-tiful they are," he said, offering me some.

"If they are that yellow-orange color, that means the apricots contain sulfur-based preservatives," I noted.

My answer surprised him. "That's impossible—I bought them in a health food store," he retorted, handing me the package.

I read through the list of ingredients and discovered an "E223" (a European code for a sulfur-based preservative). I said, "You see, that is a sulfite which allows dried fruit to keep its color. Without this E223, the apricots would have naturally turned a dark brown color, which wouldn't keep them from being delicious, because they are naturally sun-dried! Try buying packaged grated carrots in a supermarket. Forget them for a week in the fridge, and then have a look at them. If they are still beautifully or-ange, check the packaging—you're sure to find E220 to E227 sulfites."

These preservatives have given birth to paradoxes, like the handy pre-cut carrots. They're excellent for your health in their natural state, but they become toxic if you add preservatives to them. When you wake up with a headache, would you ever think of the carrots you ate the night before? Also be careful with those peanuts, almonds, hazelnuts, or cashew nuts you may be served with your drink. If they don't contain sulfites, they've been sprayed to keep their color and freshness. If you wake up feeling low the next morning, don't necessarily incriminate the alcoholic drink!

Be particularly careful with the sulfites you find in:
- frozen food products that would normally turn black in time: for example, cabbage, carrots, and potatoes;
- dried fruit, yellow raisins, apricots;
- applesauce, mayonnaise.

The food colorings used to treat the surface of citrus fruits are less toxic but not very healthy either, especially since they penetrate into the fruit and can't be washed off, even when you scrub the fruit under running water. These additives are known as "systemic products": they get inside the food and washing is ineffective to remove them.

Which foods and beverages are best?

- All kinds of *juice,* especially fresh grapefruit juice (half a glass before breakfast) and lemon or lime juice (just a little bit at the bottom of a glass with some water). If you want fruit juice containing all its natural qualities, it's best to make it fresh. If you don't have time, just eat the whole fruit.
- *Fruits,* the best of which are mango, berries (some of the best sources of antioxidants), papaya, guava, white peaches, and fresh pineapple.
- *Vegetables,* particularly bitter greens such as endive, escarole, and dandelion greens (which enhance the functioning of the liver), mache or lamb's lettuce (which is very rich in omega-3 oils), artichokes (fight cholesterol build-up), red radishes and black radish, and the king of them all, fennel.

- *Farm egg yokes and organic buttermilk* are good supplements.
- Also eat things that are slightly *sour*. Your stomach won't mind, because it is naturally highly acidic: remember, it produces hydrochloric acid, so it protects itself naturally from this acid. Slightly acid foods are much less acid than the stomach's natural secretions.

Life would be very sad if we had to stick to a strict diet all the time. Keep a balance, enjoying a rich and appetizing dish and a glass of wine once in a while. If you feel you've overdone it, go back to curative foods and plenty of water the next day.

To be consumed with moderation

Alcohol (wine, champagne, beer)
Cream, especially cooked (because it creates thyramin, which
    has an effect on the nervous system and stimulates stress)
Cheese
Cooked fats
Chocolate (we are not all equal before chocolate!)

Most vegetables have a beneficial stimulating effect on the liver, as long as they haven't been sprayed too much with toxins and are not over-cooked. Served raw or cooked *al dente,* vegetables are an aid to digestion. But if you remain attentive and keep a healthy lifestyle, don't worry about enjoying a little "naughty" treat on occasion. It's good to be a gourmet!

From a psychological point of view

- Focus on your positive attributes, without becoming arrogant or a megalomaniac. It's excellent gymnastics for the mind and keeps your liver in good health.
- Go back to the best of your experiences and extract your qualities and aptitudes from them. Recall happy events, good decisions you made, particularly enjoyable holidays, positive people who like you, successes you achieved at

work, pleasant physical sensations (sunbathing, swimming in the sea, sports, etc.). All this will help you regain or maintain your self-confidence.

- Cultivate a feeling of self-esteem and self-respect, without exaggerating, in order to acquire inner strength and radiance. Reconnect with the power of evaluating and choosing your life in full conscience and freedom, assisted by your own thoughtful reflection and the advice of trusted people.
- Seek out people with a positive attitude, whose passions and love of life will rub off on you. Avoid people who bear the misery of the world on their backs.
- Don't forget that even through our failures or what seem like unimportant acts, we can always come to good and positive realizations.

Cholesterol and the Liver

Cholesterol is found in almost all our organs. It is present in most of our hormones and contributes to the formation of others. Unfortunately, it also plays a role in forming the plaque that causes atherosclerosis (narrowing of the arteries), a condition which eventually can provoke heart attacks. This is why cholesterol has been demonized for so long. Considered merely for its negative qualities, it has terrified everyone. People complained about their cholesterol level, and doctors were set on reducing it more than necessary. Medical research has made progress in this area: we are now much more familiar with cholesterol and slightly less afraid of it. We know that our body needs it, and we also know how to differentiate between the "good" (high-density lipoprotein, or HDL) and the "bad" (low-density lipoprotein, or LDL) types of cholesterol. Doctors remain vigilant and carefully monitor their patients' cholesterol levels. An excess of the bad cholesterol that accumulates in the arteries is a risk factor we can control by living a healthy life and following a low-fat diet, not smoking, participating in the right kind of sports, and losing excess weight.

Cholesterol is present in the blood, the tissues, and all the liquids within our organism. It contributes to producing bile, sexual hormones (estrogen, testosterone, and progesterone), vitamin D, and more. Our liver synthesizes three-quarters of our cholesterol. The rest comes from food, mainly from butter, eggs, cheese, cream, and meat.

The Good and the Bad

The distinction between "good cholesterol" and "bad cholesterol" is practical, but it is an oversimplification. When it comes to cholesterol, we're not sure of anything yet! There may be good in the bad and bad in the good.

Cholesterol is transported in the blood via two different means, LDL and HDL. Both are proteins. LDL carries the cholesterol from the liver to the tissues—indeed, all tissues need cholesterol for their formation and maintenance (nerves, muscles, skin, organs). If there is too much cholesterol in this circuit, the cells don't absorb it anymore; it stays in the blood and attaches itself to the walls of blood vessels. When it stagnates cholesterol becomes oxidized, thickens, and blocks veins and arteries. HDL transports cholesterol from the tissues to the liver. playing an opposite role: it cleans the blood vessels.

The risks have been well publicized. The cholesterol that settles on the inner walls of the blood vessels forms patches of fat which end up obstructing blood circulation. A poorly irrigated organism is in danger. The risks include cardiovascular disease; obstruction of blood vessels in the brain; obstruction of the coronary arteries (heart attack); glaucoma and other types of sclerosis of the arteries in the retina; paralysis; and high blood pressure.

How to Avoid Cholesterol Build-Up

From a physical point of view

- Practice some kind of sport regularly. Whatever it may be, it will only have an effect on fat if you practice for at least half an hour.
- Maintain a healthy weight.

From a nutritional point of view

- Avoid eating too much fat: butter, fried oils, fried foods, cold cuts, fatty meats (such as rib steak), milk products (especially cheese and cream), chocolate, cakes, and pastries.
- Eat plenty of fruits and vegetables. They almost all have an antioxidant effect, to varying degrees. They slow down or prevent saturated fatty acids from clogging up our arteries with cholesterol. Certain fruits and vegetables contain fiber that latches on to the cholesterol and biliary acids and helps eliminate them. Another positive role they play is to slow down the assimilation of simple carbohydrates and help the pancreas do its job. So eat lots of fiber-rich fruits and vegetables—they are very good for your health: eggplant, carrots, celery, cabbage, turnips, onions, leek, oranges, grapefruit, tangerines, apricots, and broccoli, to name a few.
- Don't forget vitamins. You can find them naturally in foods and beverages. They are indispensable to growing children and throughout life to maintain our homeostasis, the healthy balance among all our bodily functions. Vitamins are powerful antioxidants. Two of the most beneficial ones are vitamins C and E. Without doubt, C is the most important vitamin. It can be found in citrus fruits, parsley, cabbage, peppers, radishes, kiwis, strawberries, watercress, etc. The other important antioxidant, vitamin E, can be found in almonds hazelnuts, avocados, and olive and canola oil (a subtle mix of both is excellent), among other foods.
- Choose your oils well. Prefer extra-virgin, cold-pressed olive oil, which contains antioxidants and other protective properties in the form of phenols and essential fatty acids. Canola oil also contains essential fatty acids, with a very

good balance of omega-3 and omega-6. As an added bonus, canola is one of the least expensive oils on the market.

- It is good to eat fish such as salmon, mackerel, and sardines for their healthful fatty acid content and protein. All foods that benefit the liver will help control cholesterol levels.

From a psychological point of view

- Avoid stressful situations, because stress can be an aggravating factor that raises our level of bad cholesterol. The exact mechanisms for this have not been determined, but researchers conjecture that stress encourages the body to produce more energy in the form of fatty acids and glucose. The liver must then produce and secrete more LDL cholesterol so that these substances can be transported to the other tissues of the body. Another possible contributor to higher cholesterol levels is the body's lowered ability to rid itself of excess cholesterol when highly stressed. A third consideration is the fact that stress triggers a number of inflammatory processes which increase cholesterol production.
- Try to perform your activities calmly. We often feel an inner tension deep inside, as if a rope were stretched inside our body, in our chest, around the heart and esophagus. Imagine this rope and try to relax it, from top to bottom—imagine it loosening up, waves calming down, mountains turning into hills, hard things becoming soft…. You can do this exercise of the imagination standing or lying down.
- Educate your children early on. They are deeply influenced by commercials they see on TV. Unfortunately, these commercials are well-made and persuasive: you'll grow tall and gorgeous, for example, if you eat chocolate

bars. Let's teach our children the truth: manufacturers make these ads for the purpose of selling, and these products are not good for people, especially growing children. You shouldn't totally ban sweet things, just reduce the frequency of allowing junk foods in the diet. Introduce as many fruits and vegetables as possible, early on. In Europe we have a varied diet, and this is great. Our children should keep up this tradition, but it's up to us to pass on our culinary culture to them.

• Early screening is recommended in families with a genetic risk for liver disease.

11

The Stomach and the Duodenum: Our Social Self

The stomach is the largest part of the digestive system. The food we swallow stops there long enough to be reduced to chyme (consisting of partially digested food, water, hydrochloric acid, and various digestive enzymes). The duodenum is located at the junction between the stomach and intestine, forming the initial portion of the small intestine. It prolongs digestion in the stomach and connects to the next phase of digestion in the small intestine. Although separated by the pylorus (a gate-keeper valve), the stomach and the duodenum are linked by the same digestive mechanism. The pyloric sphincter opens to let food into the duodenum, after it has been mixed with the gastric juices in the stomach. The duodenum receives the secretions produced by the liver, pancreas, and stomach—about five quarts a day.

From the digestive point of view, the duodenum is closer to the intestine, but from the emotional point of view, it's connected to the stomach. The stomach and duodenum generally react to the same emotional impulses—specifically, those connected to our relationships; in other words, the emotions that represent "me in relation to others." A hierarchy seems to exist between the two organs: A simple problem affects the stomach, while a more complex problem will involve the duodenum.

How the Stomach and Duodenum Work

The Stomach: A Grinding Pouch

This pouch, located below the ribs to the left, can contain up to one and a half quarts of food and liquid. The stomach secretes a mucus that protects its inner mucous membrane from corrosive elements and from its own acidity; it also produces and secretes up to two and a half quarts of gastric juices per day, including hydrochloric acid, which kills most of the bacteria we ingest. The sight, smell, and taste of food and drinks, or even thinking or talking about a particular dish, can call forth the secretion of gastric juices. Tea, coffee, cola, and alcohol stimulate the stomach's secretion and evacuation functions.

The stomach blends and pre-digests food then ejects it into the duodenum, in a particular order: first the carbohydrates, then the protein, and finally the fats, which are kept in the stomach up to six hours for maximum digestion and assimilation. The stomach also helps assimilate trace elements, such as vitamin B12 and iron.

The stomach is capable of absorbing water. During heat waves, you'll notice that after having a drink, you'll start sweating immediately. When the body needs water it activates the nervous system to quickly use the water that is ingested. This has to do with the stomach's connection with the vagus nerve. In this case it is not toxins you're eliminating, but water and minerals the body didn't have time to filter. It's also becoming an infamous fact that the stomach absorbs aspirin, and this can cause bleeding and ulcers if you take too much.

The Duodenum: A Cocktail Shaker

The duodenum plays a more sophisticated role in the digestive system than the grinding and chemical breakdown performed by the stomach. The duodenum is a very active organ, both mechanically as well as metabolically, since it serves to further process the material from the stomach (the chyme). The cells that line the duodenum secrete specialized hormones, which regulate the secretion of pancreatic juices and the emptying of the gallbladder and flow of bile into its lumen. Furthermore, these hormones can control the secretion of hydrochloric acid as well as the release of other enzymes into the upper gastrointestinal tract. The duodenum is the site where both bile (from the gallbladder) and pancreatic juice (from the pancreas) enter the gastrointestinal tract. Digestion is continued by the enzymes that are secreted by the duodenum's own cells, as well as enzymes contained within the bile and pancreatic juice which enters the duodenum at its mid portion. The duodenum tends to function like a cocktail shaker—with to-and-fro motion it mixes the chyme with the enzymes within its lumen.

Absorption of vitamins, minerals, and other nutrients begins in the duodenum. Once chyme enters the duodenum, its acidity is neutralized by the alkaline juices from the pancreas and bile in preparation for further digestion and absorption lower along the small intestine. There is a specialized muscle at the junction of the stomach and duodenum called the pyloric sphincter, which prevents this material from regurgitating back into the stomach.

When the Stomach Isn't Working as well as It Should

Recall that the purpose of this book is to make you aware of symptoms which indicate dysfunction, by describing in plain language some of the little signals that could make you think that your stomach (in this case) is not in perfect shape, and that it may be time to act. Of course, if that is the case, you'll have to see a doctor. Among the signs that might alert you are the following:

- acid breath in the morning and during the afternoon;
- cramps or a burning sensation underneath your left ribs (sometimes above the navel) that appears with the rooster's crow (around 4 or 5 o'clock in the morning);
- a burning sensation that can rise up toward the esophagus and send acid reflux into the mouth;
- digestive problems, such as feeling that your stomach is heavy and never empties out, or feeling full too quickly at meals;

- pains in your back, between the shoulder blades, especially when you haven't had anything to eat;
- repeated burping that briefly gives you the impression that it relieves the tension in your stomach;
- an increase in gastric problems if you eat sweet foods or drink alcohol;
- discomfort in certain positions. When lying on your stomach, the compression of the stomach impairs your breathing and causes slight nausea. You can't keep your arms raised above your head for very long. You can't stand wearing clothes or belts that are tight at the waist.

~Stomach–Duodenum People~

The stomach represents appearances; the duodenum has more to do with our true being. The stomach reacts to our social life. Further down, the duodenum is affected by more intense emotional upheaval, closer to our inner self.

• Social stress

Social stress has a particularly heavy impact on "stomach people." The stomach is the weak link, and therefore a loss of stature or support creates even further imbalance and dis-ease for the person.

Louis, who teaches in a school that has a reputation for being difficult, goes through some serious problems: clashes with students, lack of interest on the parents' part, skepticism coming from his superiors (who don't seem to be supporting him). He feels he can't go any further, can't do any more or better. It is an unbearable sense of failure for this man, considered to be a "model teacher" who had gained the respect of his students and colleagues in his previous high school teaching job. He felt like he was falling off his pedestal: his social status was being questioned, and his career seemed to be getting shaky. At this point, the repeated sense of failure began contorting his stomach. Louis was reacting on an immediate physical level to the situations he was going through at work.

Then the situation worsens. Due to total disagreement with his superiors, Louis has to leave the school. He feels frustrated in his efforts to reach a compromise. This is a heavy blow to his self-esteem, and he has a hard time facing family and friends. His innermost self is hurt. Louis starts feeling pain during the night: "It's as if my stomach is burning me," he explains to me. He can't stand belts anymore. He burps frequently. He gets hot flushes; at other times he shivers. His complexion is pale, and he looks exhausted. It isn't that occasional situations are giving him pangs of self-doubt—by now, Louis has totally lost faith in himself. His passion for teaching and his desire to help his students get through their exams have given way to discouragement. In his own words, the teacher in him has failed, but also Louis, as an individual, feels like a failure. He wants to erase the present, can't even think of the future anymore, and starts turning back to the past.

When Louis was a child, he remembers, his father didn't have much faith in him. "I'd be surprised if you ever succeed in life," he used to say to Louis all the time. The child put every effort into proving his father wrong. He didn't want to disappoint him, and had challenged himself to be a success in his teaching career, in large part to gain recognition from his father.

His doctor prescribes tests which show a duodenal ulcer. The treatment works. But Louis still has a painful spot in his back, "a pain as if a nail were being hammered in there," he says. After examining him, I explain that this spot in his back is pain transferred from his stomach—the echo of his fear of being judged by his father. A real burden!

Transferred or transference pain is also called "projected" pain. The nerve centers in an organ have their opposite end in the spine and brain. From the spine, radiation (or nervous influx) can be directed toward the skin and muscles, causing pain. The person feels uncomfortable spots in his or her back, and sometimes even real pain. The brain is the center of emotional tensions. It will try to project as much as possible into the body to free itself from an excess of negative influx. The weak link in the body—in this case, the stomach and duodenum—will literally attract these different negative influxes (whether they be physical or psychological in origin) and create an irritation.

Manual therapy of the back and Visceral Manipulation of the duodenum, along with other allopathic medical treatment, helped Louis release a lot of his physical tension. "I feel more free and less guilty," he commented. "I think seeing a psychotherapist to work on my relationship with my father would do me good."

• *The image we project to others*

The stomach and the duodenum represent our self in relation to others, at work and in society generally. To live, we need to exist socially. And what does society ask of us? That we constantly be productive and creative, while always respecting pre-established rules. To play a satisfactory role in society requires a lot of effort. It can be difficult to find one's place and exist harmoniously in a society that tends to crush its weaker members.

The stomach is a very masculine organ. People readily say of someone that "he's gutsy," meaning he is daring in his career, or that he or she has a "strong stomach." In general, ulcers are more of a male problem, particularly in young men who have reached an age where they are building up their social status, and they feel a need to prove themselves in their career and in society. Modern women taking on more and more professional responsibilities aren't spared, either. As we will see in more detail, every one of us has a yin and a yang aspect (see pages 180–181). The hormonal balance, testosterone and estrogen levels—and whether or not symptoms such as ulcers develop—depend in large measure on our personality, our education, and the society in which we live.

• *Problems with one's superiors*

Whether we are on a payroll or have our own business or practice, we always have to account for things—the employee to his boss, the CEO to the shareholders, the independent professional to his customers or patients. We frequently have to comply or compromise when dealing with superiors. It isn't cowardice, it's a question of established rules. The main thing is to keep our dignity and therefore earn respect. If tensions get too strong, the stomach reacts. Stomach people can deal perfectly well with a superior whose qualities they value, but not if the superior doesn't respect the team.

• "What I do and not what I am"

In our work and function, we're judged on the basis of facts and accomplishments. Generally, these are concrete criteria. We are asked to show what we have accomplished, rather than who we are.

Jean-Claude is a craftsman, and he has two employees. "You see," he says to me during a consultation, "I would never go away on vacation with my best worker. He is competent and efficient, but I don't like him as an individual." The funny thing is that I also treat his employee for back problems, and he thinks exactly the same of his boss.

• Appearances

In a more or less conscious way, we all build our own self-image in relation to our social front. We want to play our role, hold our rank, find our place.... A teacher giving a class is actually playing a role. You could almost say that it isn't he or she who is giving the class, but that "other person," the one who studied to become a teacher, the one who earned the appreciation and recognition of his or her students.

There was a socially brilliant and imposing teacher whose pupils were terrified of him. But as soon as he got home, he would turn into a subservient child. And his wife treated him that way, without any respect: "Put on your scarf, you're going to catch a cold" or "You're a real child!" He showed not the slightest sign of rebellion. In fact, this teacher suffered from the discrepancy between his social role and his role within his own family, where his real nature was to be weak. He acted the strong man with his students to hide his fear.

• The power of extroversion

Extroversion is what motivates us to meet other people, to get to know them, to show them we're here, to convince them. Extroversion can be natural or forced. Some shy people put on an extroverted attitude to counter their timidity. Conversely, children who were naturally extroverted and then stifled by a strict education tend to repress their true nature. Sometimes we go against our true personality and play a role to try to convince someone.

• Heightened intolerance to frustration

Stomach people who haven't achieved their goals will feel very frustrated not only with their personal plans but also with other people. It manifests in the form of stomach cramps, heartburn, and spasms. There are many pitfalls on the road to building one's career and social success. There is often good reason to feel frustrated!

• Poor self-esteem

Poor self-esteem, like other attitudes we've looked at, falls in the "too much" or "too little" category. People who overestimate situations and their own abilities set themselves up for failure, not only in their career but in their relationships with other people, who will often say, "Who does he think he is?" Rejection is only a few feet away. People who underestimate themselves will act shy and restrained, always below their potential. They are usually hampered by the weight of their education.

• Lack of self-confidence in childhood

The child we were built the adult we are. Children who lost or never had confidence in their parents, or in their own self, develop poor self-esteem. Once they become adults, depending on the other ingredients that make up their character and on how they develop, they will have a tendency either to overestimate or underestimate themselves. A father (or the man playing the father role) who oozes success will necessarily awaken admiration in his child, who will constantly strive to become the father's equal. According to the child's character, this can be an excellent catalyst or a huge hurdle leading to withdrawal and resignation. The need for recognition and power in stomach people usually implies a conflicted relationship with the father and a need to take revenge for a frustrated childhood.

• To have "guts" or a "strong stomach"

This idiom refers to a person who can take action, plan for the future, and show boldness, determination, and courage. Stomach people only feel well when they are in constant action. Never satisfied with what they have already achieved, they want to go further, ever further. The opposite of liver people (who turn back to the past), stomach people look ahead. They concentrate on the future, which keeps them from dwelling on themselves. They always have a new project. We all know that when we are absorbed by many different tasks and activities, we don't have time to think of ourselves. Living in the future in this way could be interpreted as a headlong flight, but also as a therapy that allows us to temper the deep-seated anxiety which haunts and hinders us.

To avoid failure, stomach people are overactive, always bubbling, looking for solutions and ideas. They become very creative, which can be the positive expression of anxiety. They feel and want to be responsible for everything. For better or for worse, they even create extra responsibilities for themselves which add to their workload. For example, they'll go to the office on Sunday or take work along on vacation. This kind of excitement can even turn into paranoia. They so much want to convince and succeed that they sometimes feel aggressive or the opposite (as if someone is aggressive against them), misunderstood, and unloved. They can't stand people criticizing them or being unwilling to follow their actions and ideas. This heightened need to be in full motion all the time, to surpass themselves and plan for the future, can sometimes trigger bouts of aggression in the stomach person, directed just as much toward themselves as toward other people. Aggression stimulates our cortisol level, which increases acidity in the stomach.

• Marked ambition

Because the stomach and duodenum are closely linked to our need for social recognition and the efforts we make to obtain a position of standing in society, these organs represent the image we want to show other people. If we don't succeed, it can be painful! Ambition is a means toward self-realization. But when it becomes an end in itself, it can turn against us dangerously, especially in the event of failure. If ambition is accompanied by undue arrogance, beyond the satisfaction of a well-performed task, the consequences can be even more serious. To be ambitious for oneself is a positive thing, but to be so "against" others is destructive.

• Seductive

Stomach people like to play the game of seduction. They tend to use their charm more for the pleasure of success than out of true interest in the other person. It's often a social game. Be on your guard with such people! Someone who likes to attract, to charm, to convince, and to succeed generally tends to be jealous of those who surpass them in some way. Chronic jealousy affects the stomach and the heart.

• Unstable

In their whirlwind of conquests, stomach people can be very generous, either in a truly spontaneous and unselfish way or out of a desire to show their power. It depends on the circumstances and the people involved. They can go from arrogance to humility in a flash—strong with those weaker than them, weak with the stronger! They can also shift between egotism and altruism. Egotism is hard for others to bear; altruism meant to seduce is as well. Victims feel resentful once they realize that they've been led on in a flirtatious game. And the person who played the game doesn't always feel too comfortable with his or her conscience.

• Fear of and an inability to bear failure

Stomach people have an intense need to feel supported in everything they do. They devote a lot of energy to charming and convincing others. If they don't succeed in this, they immediately feel that they are a failure. In fact, they are afraid of failure and have a very hard time with it. These are people caught in a dilemma between being a big shot and being a happy human being—with a touch of paranoia. By always wanting to impress everybody and to succeed, people who need to be center stage all the time end up creating a gap between themselves and others. They withdraw and feel misunderstood, unaccepted, disliked. Sometimes this occurs for no reason. Their friends and family circles, who are not necessarily driven by the same kind of ambition or motivations, simply don't care to follow them or to bear that kind of pressure.

• From feeling powerful to self-deprecation

The stomach is connected with our need for success and recognition. If circumstances shift such that the stomach person has lost some of their standing and power, they are gravely affected. Bernard started a very successful computer business and bought a beautiful home that he was very proud of—a tangible sign of success. The grand tour of the property was a ritual that every new guest had to go through. Then Bernard was hit by a severe economic crisis. He could no longer honor all his orders and had to lay off half of his staff. He sold the house and went back to live in an ordinary apartment. When he came to see me, he was suffering from a sore spot in his back and heartburn that got worse in the early morning. Indeed, I could feel the painful spot in his back, between the shoulder blades, toward the left. There was also abdominal pain above the navel.

In general, it is better to let patients express their problems than to ask them abrupt questions—especially men, who are shyer and have a harder time letting go. "Your stomach is tense, and I have a feeling it's not only your stomach," I said to Bernard. Then he told me of his misfortune. I knew that it was important for him to understand the relation between his stomach, which was expressing his feeling of failure, and the pain in his back. I explained, "The stomach and the muscles between the shoulder blades are connected to the same nerve centers. When the stomach gets irritated, the muscles go through spasms and cause blockage, which sends the pain back to the stomach. It's a question of the cat biting its own tail!"

It was useful to add a bit of advice: "When you feel those pains, don't try to brush them off. On the contrary: observe them, even add on to it by saying to yourself: 'It's true, it burns, it really hurts, it feels like it's tearing me apart….' The pain will become more and more specific and clear. Then put the palm of your hand on the sore spot and start thinking the opposite: 'In any case, it's no catastrophe, I'm not in danger.' Concentrate your breathing into the palm of your hand, and little by little, the pain will let off and you'll feel more and more at peace." Visceral manipulation along with breathing exercises, relaxation, and overall physical exercise eased the pain Bernard was experiencing. Understanding his pain did the rest of the job and definitely removed the "emotional nail" he had in his back. Bernard showed great interest in understanding and breaking down the system behind his pain. More and more at ease with his body and mind, he was able to reorganize his life. He gave up computers and went into air conditioning, which worked out well for him.

• *Spontaneous anger*

When something makes us angry, either we react immediately and express our anger (for example, by shouting or gesturing) or we repress it and don't let anything show. Impulsive anger affects the stomach. We feel a tightness or a burning sensation at the moment we express our anger physically, verbally, or through gestures. Suppressed anger transfers to the liver, and in particularly intense cases, the spleen.

• *"That sticks in my craw"*

We often need time to "digest" or get over strong annoyances. We'll say, "I'll have to wait for it to blow over" or "It will take a while for me to get over this." But in some cases things get "stuck" somewhere in our body's memory or our mind. We use expressions such as "That sticks in my craw," "I have a knot in my stomach," "What they did to me is hard to swallow." Vexation affects the stomach, whereas small annoyances affect the gallbladder.

How to Take Care of the Stomach

From a physical point of view

Stop smoking: whose friend can tobacco be? Mixed in with saliva, it becomes particularly toxic for the stomach.

In general, the stomach reacts positively to manual therapy (Visceral Manipulation) when we work on both the emotional and the visceral factors. A person with stomach problems is often active, even hyperactive.

Physical exercise is essential with this type of symptom, in order for the excess energy to be spent somewhere other than in the stomach. It is best to choose activities that will tire you out: cycling, running, long walks, cross-country skiing, and so on.

From a nutritional point of view

- Avoid taking in cold substances. Cold has a tendency to block the stomach and give it spasms, which prevents it from emptying properly. If you have a sensitive stomach, don't start meals with a cold dish. Hot soup is better. Eating it as a first course will relax your stomach. Asians know this, and they love soup for lunch as well as dinner. Some people even have it at the end of a meal, which is still beneficial for relaxing the stomach, just not as much as when you have it at the start of a meal.
- Chew your food thoroughly to help your stomach break it down more easily. Saliva contains enzymes which aid digestion and help us assimilate vitamins and minerals.
- Avoid sugar (for instance, adding it to your beverages or foods). It increases acidity, especially on an empty stomach. The worst times to consume sugar are at the end of the morning or in the afternoon (when the stomach is typically empty).
- Also avoid fatty foods: they aren't good for your stomach and increase acidity.
- Don't overuse aspirin and anti-inflammatory medicine. They prevent proper functioning of the protective mucus on the walls of the stomach. If you have stomach problems or an ulcer, stay away from them.

Should you eliminate acid foods from your diet? It is usually advised. But sometimes they can be beneficial. The stomach is immersed in juices more acid than most of the foods we eat. Certain acid substances help the stomach eliminate. The juice of a whole lemon may be too much for your stomach, but two or three drops in a glass of lukewarm water will help it to empty out. Of course, if you are sensitive, don't drink it on an empty stomach, at the beginning of a meal, or during the night. Stomach acids are produced in cycles: If you wake up around 2 or 3 a.m., you'll feel it more.

Foods that the "stomach person" should avoid

Lemon and vinegar (except in small quantities), oranges, sugar, chocolate, alcohol, salt, spices, garlic. To have a piece of chocolate and a bit of alcohol before going to bed is the worst thing for an acid stomach. Alcohol increases stomach acidity and causes acid reflux in the esophagus during the night.

From a psychological point of view

Stomach people are often active or even hyperactive. To prove their worth to other people, they set themselves challenging goals that aren't always within the limits of reason. There are different techniques to help them calm down a bit:

- doing "tiring out" exercise that helps them get rid of their excess energy: bicycling, running, going on long walks, cross-country skiing, windsurfing;
- practicing combat sports (martial arts), which help them temper impulses and increase self-control;
- practicing tai-chi, yoga, or relaxation.

However, their need for action is so strong that stomach people might get bored quickly. Often they return home in the evening exhausted from the day's activity. They need support from their family and friends. To say to them, "You're overdoing it, you can't keep up that pace forever" will be perceived as a negation of their work and commitment. Before they fall onto the couch, a bit of physical exercise is advisable. For instance, the simple act of going on a short walk will help them eliminate excess tension they accumulated throughout the day. Otherwise, these tensions may turn into insomnia during the night.

In serious cases, therapy can be useful to help stomach people realize why they have such a need for social recognition and why they try to lose themselves in hyperactivity. Let's not forget that the more we do, the less time we spend thinking of ourselves.

12

The Pancreas and the Spleen: Severe Emotional Shock Absorbers

From an emotional point of view, it is hard to distinguish the spleen from the pancreas, whereas on a physiological level, they have very different functions.

How They Work

The Pancreas

This oblong gland, about eight inches long, is located on the left side of the abdomen, behind the stomach. The pancreas has two functions, digestive and endocrinal:

- It secretes the enzymes we need to digest carbohydrates and fats, helping us use and transform proteins.
- It produces about one and a half quarts of pancreatic juices (for digestion) per day, which is disproportionate to its weight.
- It produces the hormones, glucagon, and insulin, which regulate our blood-sugar level. Glucagon increases it and insulin reduces it. Diabetes involves an imbalance of the two.

The Spleen

This organ is located laterally beneath the left-side ribs. It weighs no more than seven ounces. The spleen's circulatory system links it to the liver, the pancreas, and the entire body. Its functions include the following:

- It destroys red blood cells and platelets that we no longer need;
- It filters the blood and is actually a blood reserve, helping renew the precious liquid (indeed, one percent of our red blood cells die every day and need to be replaced)—the spleen can even produce red blood cells;
- It plays an important role in our immune system, defending our body against viruses, bacteria, parasites, and germs.

Amazingly enough, we can live without a spleen, although it appears to fill many functions. When the spleen has to be removed, the bone marrow will produce more red and white blood cells to compensate for the absent spleen. It will take over most of the immune defense system, thanks to the lymphocytes. From the physiological point of view, the spleen has not yet revealed all its secrets to us.

When the Pancreas and Spleen Don't Work as well as They Should

When the pancreas flashes a warning signal:

- We feel a desire to eat sweet or fatty foods as well as meat.
- We are thirsty for no apparent reason, or hungry just after eating.
- Drinking alcohol exhausts us. This is a sign that both the liver and the pancreas are having problems.
- We have digestive troubles, especially after eating fatty or sweet foods.
- We feel unwell due to poor digestion, one to three hours after meals: fatigue, nausea, sweating.
- We can't stand strong smells, such as a heady perfume or the scent of cooked cabbage.
- We feel a pain in our back, in the left shoulder blade and shoulder, without having hurt ourselves in any way.
- Some people can suffer from loosening of the teeth.

And when it's the spleen:

- We become noticeably pale and our lips are white.
- We are subject to ear, nose, and throat (upper respiratory) and sometimes lung infections. The slightest little bang causes black and blue marks. The gums tend to bleed.
- Tests show an iron deficiency. Bodywork practitioners will feel the presence of small ganglions in the armpits, behind the collarbones, and in the groin.
- There is severe fatigue, as with kidney dysfunction.
- During physical effort, there can be a side pain on the left. Around the ages of eleven or twelve, children often get that kind of cramp in their side when they run. It's an age where the immune system is undergoing deep transformation, and a time when appendicitis can occur. The spleen becomes enlarged and pulls at the diaphragm. When we're running, the diaphragm increases its mobility and pulls the spleen, which is what causes the side pain.
- After physical effort, we have a hard time recuperating.

~Pancreas-Spleen People~

In patients with illnesses linked to the spleen and the pancreas, I've had the opportunity to observe that these two organs are hard to separate on an emotional level. There are a few subtle differences, though. The pancreas and spleen react to serious events, which can upset a person for life, from childhood into old age. They absorb the most severe shocks.

• Unbearable stress

Stress and extreme shock can cause a dysfunction in the pancreas, even to the degree of causing the onset of diabetes. There are several types of diabetes, with the most well-known form called sugar diabetes. This illness is linked to insufficient secretion of insulin, or an incapacity to properly use the insulin produced by the pancreas, causing poor regulation of the blood sugar. Its level increases in the blood and urine (hyperglycemia).

The person drinks constantly, urinates frequently, eats too much, and often suffers from skin problems, infections, circulatory troubles, eye and kidney problems.

As a result of its role in insulin secretion, the pancreas is in charge of regulating the amount of sugar in the blood and body when this level is too high. When blood sugar is low the pancreas releases the hormone glucagon, which signals the liver to release glucose.

Marguerite, a relatively young grandmother of three, particularly adores her seven-year-old granddaughter. "That little girl is just like me. I feel like I'm seeing myself at her age," she likes to say. One day she picks up the little girl to take her to the movies. During the trip, the little girl is sitting calmly on the back seat. A truck driving just ahead of them stops suddenly. A cement beam flies out of the truck and lands on Marguerite's car, on the right side, where the little girl is seated. She is killed on the spot. Sorrow, anguish, and guilt assail Marguerite. A week after the accident, she contracts diabetes.

In Marguerite's case, there was no indication of diabetes in her family history. The trigger was the indescribable stress she went through. She has been a diabetic dependent on insulin ever since.

• Unaccepted deaths

In the case of bereavement, a heart-rending separation, a natural catastrophe, a particularly terrible accident, a terrorist attack, and other tragic events, we have to face up to and reflect upon the possible meaning of our suffering and the event itself, and work on acceptance. This psychological process can be gone through alone or with the help of friends and/or a therapist. The spleen and pancreas react to deaths that have not been accepted. Another of my patients, Marie-Christine, lost her husband and can't help saying to anyone who'll listen, "It's not fair! We were such a close couple! I'll never be able to accept it." A few months after his death, she developed leukemia.

The spleen and pancreas have close vascular connections. When one of the two organs is hit, the other one is often affected too. In the case of Marie-Christine, the shock hit her spleen, causing a breakdown of her immune system. She realized later that having refused to accept her husband's death had left her body totally off balance. Today she has been cured of the leukemia. The medical treatment worked, of course, but the psychological help she got was a determining factor. "It's strange," she explains, "I felt the exact moment my head helped my body." Because Marie-Christine succeeded in accepting her husband's death, her body felt better.

"To overcome one's grief" does not mean that the emotional shock has been erased, but that the loss of the loved one has been accepted and integrated into one's life path and no longer triggers physical disability.

• Meeting with one's own mortality

Our civilization, with its cult of youth and idealized appearances, of conspicuous consumption and continuously "changing channels" to seek the new, usually keeps us too busy to think about death. We hide our head in the sand like an ostrich! Although we know it is inevitable, we put off as long as possible thinking about death deeply and seriously. Going through physical trauma, getting mugged, or experiencing a narrow escape from death are huge shocks for people who closed their eyes to the fact until then. One often hears the maxim "To live a successful life means to accept the idea of dying." This thought may seem restrictive, but it can help us realize the task that lies before us. If we have never thought about the inevitability of death and we're suddenly confronted with it, the spleen and pancreas react and stop performing their respective functions properly. The person will have repeated infections, will be very tired even when at rest, their body will have trouble regulating its blood sugar, and they will feel unquenchable thirst.

• Being confronted with physical violence

It would be ideal, of course, to live in a peaceful society where everyone attends to their own business in harmony with others; where relationships within the family, at work, as well as socially develop free of clashes. Unfortunately, reality is often very different. Some people experience extreme violence. To be subject to the violence of an individual or a group of people hurts us in our deepest reaches, on all levels. These unacceptable and intolerable situations provoke immediate physical reactions such as vomiting, diarrhea, and trembling. They resonate in our weaker points (our weak link) or in the organs that are particularly receptive to violence, such as the spleen and pancreas. These organs will act like time bombs (repeated infections, poor glycemia regulation, unquenchable thirst).

• *An unsatisfying life*

A person who is stifling a large part of his or her self in order to do what they feel they should for their family could wind up with pancreatic challenges. Nicolas married young, and his wife was a girl from abroad who did not want to live in France. He left his country, his family, and his friends to be with her. He initially had a hard time with this total uprooting from his home, and then Nicolas seemed to adapt to his new life. Yet several years after his "exile," for no apparent reason, he contracted an inflammation of the pancreas. Leaving his wife and children for a while, he came back to France to tend to his health. I was among the doctors and therapists he saw. He told me several times, "I'm not living the life I wanted—I made a mistake from the start. I tried to adjust my life to the decision I had made, but I never stopped regretting this choice." Being back in France forced this crucial dilemma on Nicolas: to live in France or to live with his family. I don't know what the outcome was—I never saw him again. In any case, it was very hard for me to offer a solution to so personal a problem.

• *A crushed or stolen childhood*

Childhood memories should be full of tenderness, affection, and feelings of being protected. But sometimes—for family or social reasons, negligence, perversion, distorted behavior, etc.—these memories are the opposite: humiliating, terrifying, violent and devastating. According to the situation and the child's character, some people react with fatalism, while others react with rage and determination.

Chantal is in her forties. She always saw her mother in serious depression: ups and downs, suicide attempts, stays at the hospital, chronic alcoholism.

As a child she was spared nothing. She tells of her difficulties but confesses, "Despite it all, I always loved my mother." Chantal complains of abdominal pains. A scan show shows numerous calcification spots in her pancreas, devoid of any physiological cause, but perfectly understandable with regard to her life story.

Zooming In on the Spleen

Some reactions are more specifically linked to the spleen, although the division with the pancreas is an extremely fine line. The following traits could apply to anyone with a weakened spleen, or to someone who is not a spleen person but develops problems with this organ.

• Deep pessimism

This quality associated with the spleen is not so much the pessimistic reaction to a specific event, but an all-encompassing, continual pessimism, due to an inborn or acquired dysfunction of the spleen. It makes some spleen people the kind of person who sees everything painted black, always focusing on the bad side of things. Whenever they begin any endeavor or action, they'll say, "It won't work, I have bad luck, it's always been that way, there's no reason for things to change." It is exhausting for people around them, who eventually give up after trying for too long to infuse some winning spirit into their friend.

• Deep sadness

Like the pervasive pessimism described above, sadness is ever-present in a spleen person. The person carries the weight of the world on their shoulders. That little spark that shines in the eyes has dimmed with them. Sometimes it's hard to know why. There is no more energy there. The person can be affable but lacks enthusiasm and reacts lifelessly to joys as well as to sorrows. It may seem like nothing touches them anymore, but deep down inside, they've remained sensitive. This is not the kind of person to go to if you need a bit of pepping up!

• Despair, inconsolable sorrow

When everything is going wrong, when we have no strength to react anymore, when we are overcome with dejection and despair, we are usually dealing with the aftermath of horrible and unacceptable events. If our spleen doesn't work well, we won't have sufficient energy to accept the situation, to fight and to endure. Luckily, such extreme situations are rare.

Claire and Jean were experienced mountain climbers. Almost every weekend, weather permitting, they would climb the highest mountains in Europe. One day Jean, who was the leader, fell in front of Claire, who was right behind him. She had the incredible luck not to be dragged down with him. She saw Jean hanging at the end of his rope, unconscious, until the rescue team arrived several hours later. "It was horrible," she says, "I heard his head crack." Jean did not survive the accident. Claire suffered a spleen attack that left her with pain in her abdomen and left shoulder, typical of spleen reactions.

• Devouring remorse

The spleen plays an important role in our immune system. Emotions such as remorse and despair which are connected to the spleen will gravely affect a person's health. Pierre and his family witnessed a mugging in the metro. Three individuals were beating up a man with a baseball bat, and Pierre didn't intervene. He still feels heavy remorse. Trying to justify himself, he says, "Do you realize that train or subway controllers always tell passengers not to intervene when violence occurs on the train, just to pull the alarm. Imagine yourself in this situation—what would you have done?"

Pierre struggled most with the memory of the questioning and begging look in his children's eyes, which seemed to say to him, "Why aren't you doing anything? You're an adult, you're strong, you always told us how important it is to help other people...." His family and friends are doing everything they can to help him get over his guilt feelings, assuring Pierre that they would have reacted the same way. But Pierre can't escape the haunting remorse he feels. His character has changed. He has become withdrawn, as if branded by his children's judgment of him at the moment of the violent event. Since that time, he is prone to catching infections, especially a sore throat. Remember that the spleen is a key element in our immune system.

• *Severe childhood trauma*

"We really wanted a boy." These words she repeatedly heard her parents say marred Claude's childhood. In her fifties, she admits to still being shocked by this statement, which made her feel "guilty" for being a girl. Her parents called her Claude, not Claudine or Colette—real girl's names. "It's strange," she says, "how my parents didn't even realize that they hurt and traumatized me by saying that. I am married, I have two grown children, but sometimes—for example, when I look at myself in the mirror—I can't help wondering what if, deep inside, I were really a boy?"

Claude has a real problem with her identity. Hearing one's parents repeat "We would have preferred a boy" is destabilizing, to say the least: "This leitmotif of feeling guilty for being a girl is unbearable!" Claude said. She suffered from mononucleosis, with serious consequences that lasted years: fatigue, hair loss, brittle nails, severe paleness, deficient muscles. She had to rest for two to three hours every afternoon. Finally a lymphocyte deficiency, due to impaired spleen function, was diagnosed. Thanks to the right medical treatment, Claude was cured, and she now feels much better psychologically as well. Because a physical imbalance in an organ can cause emotional and psychological disturbances, the healing of that same organ can help to correct the emotional upset. It is also true that positive work on the psychological component can facilitate healing in the associated organ. There are multiple ways to get the mountaintop of optimal health)!

How to Take Care of the Pancreas and Spleen

From a physical point of view

- Get into that habit of doing breathing exercises. Try stretching, which is an excellent way of relaxing the body and strengthening your defense system to stress.
- Boost your immune system with healthy walking and other forms of aerobic activities.

From a nutritional point of view

For the pancreas to help you "digest" stress, choose your foods well. Eat little to none of the following foods, which contain too much simple carbohydrates (sugar) for the spleen:

- sugar, honey, jam, sweetened soda
- chocolate, commercial cereals
- white bread, biscuits
- white rice
- French fries and all greasy foods
- butter, cheese
- alcohol: Beware of beer! It contains both alcohol and sugar. People who drink too much of it can develop inflammation of the pancreas.

The insulin secreted by the pancreas allows us to regulate our blood sugar. The more sweets we eat, the more insulin the pancreas produces, and the more it produces, the more the body stores fats. Today we speak of the "glycemic index" of foods, referring to how rapidly a food's sugar content is assimilated. Certain sodas (with extreme levels of high-fructose corn syrup and sugar) are at the top of the list of all foods and beverages. The simple carbohydrate (high glycemic index) content of these foods and drinks is as important as the quantity of them that we consume. For example, dark chocolate consumed as pure or close to pure cacao (the raw ingredient) has a low glycemic index, but the sugars and other added ingredients can alter it to become a high-glycemic-index food.

The best foods are fiber-containing vegetables and fruits, because they slow down the passage and assimilation of simple carbohydrates. They also lighten the burden put upon the pancreas by preventing extreme glycemic swings (ups and downs). Here are some of the higher-fiber vegetables and fruits: asparagus, broccoli, cucumbers, green beans, peas, spinach, leek, endives, garlic, cantaloupe, berries, blackcurrants, apricots, peaches, plums, watermelon, and papaya.

Patients have also felt the benefits of certain starches: whole-grain bread, brown rice, beans, lentils, tabouli, and oatmeal. Nutritionists frequently recommend fish containing a lot of omega-3 (including sardines, salmon, herring, and red mullet) and soluble fiber (pectin, gum), which is found in fruits and vegetables—these nutrients help fight off hyperglycemia attacks.

The spleen plays a little-known role in assimilating iron. To avoid deficiencies, eat foods that contain a lot of iron: calf's liver, potatoes, lentils, seafood, fish, eggs. The spleen also seems to benefit from foods containing significant quantities of magnesium, such as almonds, hazelnuts, cacao (raw chocolate), and soy.

From a psychological point of view

Much of your mental and physical health depends on the stress you have been through. If it is too heavy to bear, it's best to see a psychotherapist or psychoanalyst. Claire, whom you've already encountered in this chapter, felt guilty for having suggested that fatal climb to her husband. She saw a therapist for six years. I also helped her free the many physical tensions which her body had memorized. Today Claire has resumed mountain-climbing.

If the stress is not severe, chase away dark moods by enjoying the good things in life: your friends, hobbies, culture. Take advantage of the activities that fill you with life, love, and energy. Value people who know how to make you feel at ease. Spend time with people who are soothing and positive, and learn to say no to others. Go to the theater, the movies, do some stretching, dancing, playing music. Fix up your home: bright rooms, pictures that invite you to dream and to travel, maybe a change to the place where you sleep.

We all have an animal instinct, a sense of our den, which will make us prefer a certain spot in the kitchen, in the living room, in the bedroom. Try out different areas in a room and you'll see that you feel calmer in some spots than in others. Every human body produces and picks up an electromagnetic field. Don't think too much about it—just spend time in the places where you feel best.

13

The Intestines:
A Long and Winding Road

The intestines are by far the longest organ in the human body, about twenty-six feet in total length, including twenty-one feet of small intestine and five feet of large intestine. The intestinal mucous membrane (particularly in the small intestine) is characterized by its numerous coils, which increase the surface in contact with the chyme (food reduced to a pulp by the stomach), optimizing the absorption of nutrients. In the small intestine, there is constant movement: the chyme is re-mixed up to sixteen times a minute. The intestine molts. The cells on its inner surface are renewed every two days. It is a hypersensitive transmitter-receiver of emotions: a hundred million neurons link it to the brain—a superconnection! That is why you "feel it in your gut."

How the Intestines Work

An Absorber and Re-Absorber

Working together with the other digestive organs, the intestines absorb anything consumed that can be useful to the body. They assimilate fats and help dissolve cholesterol. By the time the chyme leaves the small intestine, most of the nutrients have been absorbed. The large intestine reabsorbs the water content of the chyme, transforming it from liquid to solid, and shaping it into feces. We mustn't forget that almost two gallons of water per day pass through the digestive system, from the mouth down to the anus. The intestines re-absorb a large part of it, passing it into the blood and lymph. This explains why suppositories (any medicine taken into the body via the rectum) are effective.

Each part of the intestine is specially designed to absorb selective vitamins or minerals. If that part of the intestine is in trouble, then you may not get those vitamins or minerals, even if the food intake or supplements provide huge quantities of it. The small intestine absorbs such vitamins as B12 and C, and minerals like magnesium and zinc. The large intestine houses more than seven hundred species of bacteria which perform a variety of functions. The large intestine absorbs some of the products formed by the bacteria inhabiting this region. These bacteria also produce small amounts of vitamins, especially vitamin K and vitamin B, for absorption into the blood. Along with the liver, the intestines are affected by the cycles of the sexual hormones. This hormone connection may be the most frequent cause of intestinal problems, particularly in women. By breaking down (pre-digesting) fats, the bile and pancreatic secretions make the intestines' job of assimilating food easier. For the intestines to function properly, the liver and the pancreas have to do their job first.

When the Intestines Don't Work as well as They Should

• Flatulence

When over-reactive or irritated, the small intestine does not break food down completely. As a result, the food makes it into the large intestine in an undigested state. There, the undigested food meets up with billions of hungry bacteria—the natural "intestinal fauna" we all have in our large intestine. These bacteria are happy to digest the food. They produce a variety of gases, including methane, hydrogen, and hydrogen sulfide. Hydrogen sulfide is the source of the odor we associate with flatulence. Wearing a belt or overly tight pants becomes a problem when the intestines are not working properly. The tightness is bearable in the morning, intolerable in the afternoon as the gases start to build up.

• A tight and tense abdomen

The intestine is a muscle that fulfills its function through an unceasing succession of contractions. When it isn't functioning well, it causes abdominal cramps.

• Morning tiredness

Morning tiredness can be an indication of a problematic intestine. "Intestine" morning tiredness is not as severe as the fatigue caused by a kidney or pancreas problem. It often comes along with a bad mood, and tends to disappear as the day goes on.

• Reflux and eructation

Tension and the presence of air in the intestines prevent the diaphragm from moving comfortably. In such cases, burping is the best way to relax the abdomen. Some people do it too often, and it becomes a kind of a tic. When the intestine pushes the diaphragm upward, the diaphragm drags the junction between the esophagus and the stomach upward. The negative pressure within the chest attracts the hydrochloric acid from the stomach toward the esophagus and causes heartburn.

• Constipation and hemorrhoids

Fecal matter that stagnates for too long in the intestinal duct hardens and becomes difficult to eliminate. For some people, the troubles of constipation become an obsession, or even a phobia. The feces that haven't been eliminated become an obstacle to proper blood and lymph circulation. They compress the veins, which can dilate and form hemorrhoids. Don't forget that the intestines' real stimulators are first the liver, and then the pancreas. In the morning, after breakfast, dilatation of the stomach and stimulation of the bile and pancreatic functions bring on the need to go to the toilet. The intestine is as accurate as a clock. Sooner is too early, later is too late! If you miss the right moment, constipation sets in.

• Diarrhea

The loose stools of diarrhea are often due to over-emotionality, which stimulates our sympathetic nervous system—the one that excites most of our organs. If you catch a cold that goes straight to your stomach you will often experience diarrhea. Watch out for constipation-diarrhea cycles, and for black feces (if you haven't eaten any licorice). Talk to your doctor about it.

• Spasms and muscular cramps

When we are mentally irritated, the long muscle that makes up the intestine can stay contracted. Blood circulation in the arteries and veins, as well as lymph circulation, are reduced, which makes it more difficult to absorb minerals and trace elements. Without these essential nutrients, muscles have a tendency toward spasms and tetany.

• Spasmophilia and fibromyalgia

These syndromes are more frequent in women. According to Drs. Curtay and Razafimbelo,[*] spasmophilia is a genetic predisposition that affects eighteen percent of the population. This condition is characterized by cramps, a tingling sensation, restlessness, and back spasms. It indicates a serious magnesium deficiency. Related to hypoglycemia, this syndrome includes anxiety, hunger, accelerated heartbeat, trembling, and perspiration. You are tired when you get up in the morning and have sudden urges to go to sleep; you feel numbness in the hands and feet. You get cramps in the calves, feet, and back; spasms in the stomach, gallbladder, or colon; headaches, dizziness, or sharp back pains. You are easily irritated, nervous, or anguished. You can almost surely diagnose this as spasmophilia. These signs vary in intensity and location. They are mostly attributed to stress, and occur at or near season changes. Besides stress, other causes may lead to spasmophilia, such as vitamin deficiency (mostly D); a lack or imbalance of minerals (calcium, magnesium, potassium, or phosphorus);

---

[*] Dr. Jean-Paul Curtay and Dr. Rose Razafimbelo, *Le Guide familial des aliments soigneurs (The Family Guide To Foods That Heal),* Paris: Albin Michel, 2005.

or a sexual hormone disorder related to glands (at the thyroid, parathyroid, or suprarenal levels).

Fibromyalgia is an extremely intense state of weakness that lasts for more than six months and resists rest. The intestinal hormone connection is one of its causes. One of the first things to do to heal spasmophilia and fibromyalgia is to treat the intestine through diet and the right kind of exercise. Fibromyalgia is more commonly encountered in the U.S. than spasmophilia. Spasmophilia actually does not exist in most English-speaking countries, as severe mineral imbalances are not as common in developed countries, and it is less and less a topic in France. There seem to be cultural reasons for this—family, media, education. For example, taking a spoonful of olive oil is effective for the gallbladder in Italy, but perhaps not in other countries. This is because Italian families believe that olive oil has strong healing and health-enhancing properties, but this may not be the dominant belief elsewhere. Whether or not something is good or bad, the placebo effect plays a large role in making it so (due to cultural and educational understanding).

• Pain in the joints

These pains particularly affect the lumbar vertebrae, the knees, and the feet. There is often a connection between a functional problem in the intestine and *hallux valgus,* better known as bunions. The relationship between the intestine and *hallux valgus* has been clinically observed (with astonishing frequency). We do not have a medical explanation for this, but it is my belief that the connection is through the femoral nerve.

• Striated and brittle nails

This symptom is also found in people who have kidney problems. It could have to do with faulty assimilation of calcium, magnesium, and zinc.

~Intestine People~

The intestine is one of the organs most prone to psychosomatic (mind-body) reactions. It is often tense, bloated, or irritated. With its network of a hundred million neurons, it is subtly and powerfully connected to the brain, whose emotional implications are often contradictory and paradoxical. These emotions are paired with physiological reactions: constipation or diarrhea. Emotional sensitivity of the intestines is greater in women.

• A great need for security and protection

"Protect me" or "I want to protect you"—that is what the intestines say. They represent our need to be protected as well as to protect. Intestine people seek security and protection, for themselves and for others. By protecting those around them, they protect themselves. The overprotective mother is a typical case—she is extremely careful to see that nothing happens to her children. She warns of every possible danger. "Watch that step! Watch out with those matches! Watch the road!" But once she has warned and protected, her doubts and anxiety come back. She seems strong and hides her frailness behind a facade. She puts on an air of self-confidence, the better to hide her anxiety.

Mothering sometimes extends beyond the children and includes the partner, who becomes a child to be protected too. Marie-Odile, a mother of five children, is an admirable woman. She runs her household masterfully. Her husband comes to see me for a very painful case of lumbago. She comes along as well. From the very first question, she's the one who answers. Of course! She manages her family outside the home just as much as inside. The interesting thing about it is that her husband doesn't seem to mind, although he knows he should be the one to answer. He accepts her intervening and even looks up to her in admiration. An intestine woman needs to be protected, but at the same time this "strong-minded" woman knows how to assert herself.

• A great need to talk

Intestine people talk a lot, sometimes to the point of logorrhea (pathologically excessive talking). Their words fill in the empty spaces that would force them to confront their deep-seated anxiety. The more anxious they are, the more they talk. Carole comes to see me for the first time. She hasn't even sat down, and she is already telling me her story.

I have to interrupt her to write out her card. "If you don't mind," I say, "I need to ask you for some basic information. What is your name?" She gives me her name and immediately goes on to tell me what happened to her the night before. She doesn't leave me a chance to get a word in edgewise—she never stops, asking questions and giving the answers herself, trying to convince me and to prove to herself that she is right. She seems to be having an entire debate all on her own. Finally noticing the astounded look on my face, she realizes the absurdity of the situation and excuses herself: "I know, I always talk too much and too fast, but I can't help it." The consultation can now begin. It isn't good to make advance judgments in my profession, but it seemed pretty obvious to me that the intestine was this patient's weak spot. This was confirmed through my questions and palpation.

• Great faithfulness

Intestine people are not only faithful in marriage—they are also faithful to associates, friends, therapists, their hairdresser, etc. They build themselves their own little safe world. This reassures them. Marie-Pierre is a typical illustration of the "intestine person." She has been coming to me for a very long time, at least once or twice a year. Every visit she brings me a croissant and a cake and puts them on my desk, saying: "Go ahead, eat them, you're too skinny and you work too hard." It's almost as if she wants to reverse the roles and make me her patient! I've often tried to recommend other practitioners to her, but she always comes back to me, saying, "You're the only one who knows how to take care of me—no one else!"

• Remarkably meticulous

An intestine person's home is spotlessly clean and tidy. She keeps her house in perfect shape. This can border on obsession or obstinacy. She can't stay seated for a minute. She has to straighten out, wash, scrub, dry. She is an active person who needs to expend her energy to feel right. Ask her to perform a task for you, and she'll do it to perfection.

• Obstinate

Active and meticulous, intestine people are also very determined. You could say that when their mind is set on something, there's no swaying them. They persevere to the point of obstinacy! For example, Martin has joined a charity that takes care of financially and psychologically distressed families. A trained lawyer, he rapidly becomes indispensable to the organization. But he and the president clash. They have opposite opinions. She doesn't want to follow his line of conduct, and he obstinately keeps trying to make her accept his way. He puts a lot of energy into it. Tension flares up repeatedly. Without any previous symptoms, suddenly Martin develops rectal bleeding. The medical diagnosis is reassuring: it is due merely to stress-related diverticula (small bulging sacs pushing outward from the colon wall). So, knowing he is not going to convince the president and that he can't give up, he decides to leave the organization rather than become upset again. His intestine relaxes, and the diverticula cause him less trouble.

• A great need to convince

Needing to convince means always needing to be right. Intestine people can't understand that other people may not want to follow their ideas or decisions. As we already know, they possess great energy. So what could be better to spend it on than their own ideas and convictions?

• Hypochondria

Hypochondriacs are constantly worried about their health. The slightest little ache or pain, and they think it's a disease. They ask everybody around them health and medical questions and are constantly on the lookout for their reactions. They seek every possible indication to confirm their fears: "I knew it, there's something seriously wrong with me, and you don't want to tell me." Their hypochondria comes in cycles; the symptoms change and therefore so does the illness. But the attitude remains the same. Their fear of disease is an obsession, and the way they project it onto their family and friends often resembles emotional black-mail. They won't hesitate to put in a little comment such as "Even if I'm sick, I always take care of you first." For hypochondriacs, the real issue isn't healing, but the attention that their ills give them.

• A tendency toward exaggeration and theatrics

Intestine people have a tendency to dramatize sad or happy events, with-out any evil intent. Usually they overdo things to reassure and convince other people, but mainly to reassure and convince themselves. When joyful, they let out their excess energy. When they are sad, they seem to say, "Don't worry about me, I'm suffering, but I'll be OK." Even those who know the intestine person well have a hard time telling the real feel-ings from the theatrics.

• Slightly obsessive

Details take on great importance. When looking too closely at the trees, one doesn't see the forest. The intestinal function becomes an obsessive problem, a phobia. The slightest travel or change in habits causes consti-pation, a real drama. Intestine people tend to exaggerate their intestinal problems, just like they do all ailments. They project their own obsession on others. If one of the children is constipated, they'll pour advice and care onto them.

• A certain rigidity

These are people with principles. For them, certain behaviors are "done" or "not done." And when something is not to be done, there's no going against the rules. It's no use trying to loosen up these rigidly principled people. They tend to educate their children in a strict manner. The same psychological rigidity is found in their meticulous habits or obsession with order and cleanliness. But if you know which button to push, you can make this kind of person bend or give in. They are so emotionally needy!

• Mood swings

Intestine people often have uneven moods. Within a few hours, or less, they can go from being in a great mood to becoming irritated over nothing. Alas, some little detail isn't quite right, and the entire picture changes. They sense somehow that their mood has swung, but they can't help being unpleasant.

• Great generosity

Intestine people like to help out. Even if they sometimes complain about getting nothing in return, they are sincerely generous. They find comfort and protection in being that way. By giving to others, they avoid feeling sorry for themselves. They like to get involved in charities or humanitarian action.

• Sensitive and thin-skinned

Intestine people are sensitive and vulnerable, and therefore susceptible to the vagaries of fortune and the insults of others. They are easily offended. We all have our weak spots that it's best not to provoke, lest we overreact. This is particularly true of intestine people. They are sensitive concerning themselves, and in regard to their loved ones. So watch what you say to them. If you make the wrong remark at the wrong time, you'll see a friendly face turn into a stiff mask, and a smile into cold anger.

• An inclination toward paranoia

When they're not at their best or something goes slightly out of sync in their schedule, intestine people are prone to thinking that they're the victim of some plot. Luckily, it's on a small scale. When they're down, they might think their family is in league against them. When they're in good health, these impressions disappear quickly. Such people desperately want others to follow what they think and do.

How to Take Care of the Intestines

From a physical point of view

- Walk as much as possible. To work properly, those twenty-six feet (approximately) of intestines need activity. Walking is excellent stimulation, helping to "stir" the contents of the intestine and to eliminate the air it contains.
- Do breathing exercises. This allows the diaphragm (the muscle that makes us breathe) to give the abdomen a massage. Do a few deep-breathing sessions with a manual therapist to learn the basic movements.
- Watch your spine. A blocked lumbar vertebra, a disc problem, a shock to the coccyx can all cause intestinal problems, particularly constipation. Have your spine looked at by a properly trained manual therapy practitioner.

From a nutritional point of view

Fermentation of foods can occur in the large intestine if the stomach and small intestine are not functioning optimally and the food is not thoroughly digested. Certain foods are known to ferment in the intestines: beans, peas, cabbage, chickpeas (a.k.a. garbanzo beans), onions, artichokes, mushrooms, leek (they contain sulfur). It's best to eat them cooked (either steamed or boiled), and changing the water once in the course of cooking. Chew them thoroughly, because the enzymes in our saliva make foods easier to digest. Certain cheeses, if they are overripe, are also candidates for fermentation.

Foods that contain too many pesticides can irritate the intestines. Get into the habit of buying at farmers' markets or health food stores, at least once a week. Larger supermarkets are beginning to carry more organic products.

Stress and the seasons also have an influence on intestinal tolerance. In women, the intestines react differently at different times in the hormonal cycle. Women are more sensitive to certain foods before their period or during menopause.

To heal and avoid constipation the best remedy is to eat fiber-rich vegetables and fruits. As we've mentioned, boiling or steaming are the healthier methods of cooking them. Choose the foods you tolerate best and that seem helpful to you among the following: leek, endives, string beans, spinach, squash, citrus fruits, grapes, bananas, fresh pineapple, rhubarb. The "Golden Globe" goes to figs—there's nothing better to activate a lazy intestine. If you are constipated, it may be useful to alternate cold and hot. Have a cup of coffee, for instance, after eating a sherbet.

From a psychological point of view

- Learn to rest and to relax. The cleaning or mowing can wait a few minutes: put on some music, lie down, relax your muscles, and let the music seep into you.
- Why run? Slow down, and you'll see how many details you missed in a person or a place, because you were going too fast.
- Try not to imagine the worst possible scenario when your wife or husband is on a trip or your children at school. Think about yourself instead.
- Learn to speak more slowly, letting other people talk. Listen to them first, and wait your turn. When you talk too much, you smother others and discourage them from speaking.

14

The Kidneys:
Two Non-Identical Twins

Physiologically speaking, the kidneys, whose function is elimination, are identical twins. But emotionally speaking, they are non-identical. Each one perceives different emotions and deals with them in its own way.

How the Kidneys Work

The left kidney and the genital system largely share the same blood and lymph circulation circuits. This probably explains why the left kidney is connected to sexuality and genitality. To treat one of these systems, you have to work on the other one too. The right kidney is more dependent upon the digestive system. Located just below the liver, it often works in close connection with it. It's the liver's outlet.

• They manage the water in our body

The human body is seventy percent water (the percentage varies throughout life—highest when we are young and typically decreasing with age). Our kidneys are in charge of maintaining that level and distributing the water throughout the body. They control our blood volume and blood pressure in close collaboration with the other organs. They keep watch over the sodium, potassium, calcium, phosphorus, and bicarbonate levels in our body.

• They eliminate our waste

The kidneys filter more than 395 gallons of blood and produce about one and a half quarts of urine per day. What a huge job! Our entire blood system gets cleaned out every twenty-four hours. The kidneys eliminate the water and salt to prevent the tissues from retaining them in excess. When they don't do their job properly, there can be a risk of edema (fluid retention and swelling). They also eliminate the waste and toxins that our cells produce. You could say that, along with the liver, the kidneys are the greatest cleaners in our body. They transform protein (mostly from meat and milk products) into urea and uric acid. They excrete certain soluble waste matter, such as nitrogenous waste, hormones, and medicines.

• They produce non-sexual hormones

The kidneys have nothing to do with the production of sexual hormones. They do, however, secrete two hormones: erythropoietin (acts on the bone marrow to increase the production of red blood cells) and calcitriol (which acts on the cells of the intestine to promote the absorption of calcium from food, and acts on the bone to mobilize calcium from the bone to the blood), as well as the enzyme renin (which has an influence on blood pressure). The kidneys also play a role in synthesizing prostaglandin (which has an influence on the uterus, the digestive system, the bronchial passages, and pain).

• Other functions

The kidneys stimulate production of red blood cells and vitamin D and help us store glucose.

When the Kidneys Don't Work as well as They Should

Early Morning Symptoms

When the kidneys have too many proteins and toxins to eliminate, or when we have an infection, the following signals are likely to be present:

- Deep fatigue that is hard to overcome.
- Sleep that brings no rest.

- Skin that marks when you pinch it.
- Rings under the eyes, and light is hard to bear.
- Swollen eyelids.
- A crumpled face, a waxen complexion.
- Hair that has no shine or shape.
- Particularly intense lumbago in the morning, subsiding in the course of the day.
- Unpleasant hunger pangs that seem to cause stomach cramps.
- A feeling of pins and needles in the feet when you get out of bed.

Persistent Symptoms

- Swollen legs and feet, sometimes even when waking up in the morning.
- Sensitivity to cold; fear of cold water.
- A need to press the thumbs or palms against the lumbar area of the spine to soothe the kidneys. This will help in the event of kidney-related lumbago, whereas it will irritate a vertebral problem.
- Variable blood pressure—usually low at the onset of kidney dysfunction and high if the problem becomes chronic.
- Pain in the lumbar area at night, whereas mechanically caused lumbago is relieved by lying down.
- Bouts of pessimism.
- Attacks of intense pain in the stomach or back, indicating the presence of stone-forming crystals (microlithiase) in the urine, excreted by the kidneys. The pain comes in short waves but is often exhausting.
- Unclear urine, with a strong smell of ammonia.

The Left Kidney

Since the genital organs' venous system is closely linked to that of the left kidney, an infection in the genital area will affect the left kidney. Practitioners who work on both systems will obtain better results. Since it works in symbiosis with the urogenital system, the left kidney echoes our sexuality and sensuality. When we speak of sexuality, we do not mean only the sexual act itself. We're talking in a wider sense about a certain potential that includes all phenomena related to the sexual instinct and its satisfaction. This is in us, even if we do not live it out. As to sensuality, we mean the person's attachment to the pleasures of the senses and to erotic sensations.

The Right Kidney

Considered the liver's outlet, the right kidney is important in filtering and eliminating waste. From an emotional point of view, the right kidney's function is to rid us of psychological overflow from the liver. So you'll find the same emotional characteristics that apply to liver people. When the liver and the right kidney are both dysfunctional, the body has very little possibility of compensating for the physical or emotional imbalance. The person will feel extremely worn out physically and psychologically and will usually require therapeutic help.

Kidney Stones

Kidney stones occur when the kidneys are no longer able to eliminate certain waste matter (comprised of salts and minerals), which then crystallizes into small hard "stones." The stones can form in the ureter or bladder, in addition to the kidneys. They are often evacuated with the urine without provoking any symptoms, but sometimes they cause intense pain when passing that feels like being stabbed with a knife.

Kidney Prolapse or "Ptosis of the Kidneys"

The kidneys, which are the chief organs of excretion, are not attached by ligaments but are held in their pockets by a wrapping of fat. This lack of supportive ligaments makes the kidneys very unstable. Furthermore, because of their high density and compactness, they are very sensitive to the shock waves caused by trauma. There can even be micro-fractures. A loose kidney is almost always found with faulty posture. The drooped thorax obliterates the forward thrust of the ribs and relaxes the diaphragm, thus pushing the liver downward on the kidney to the right. Because of this pressure the protective fat is rapidly lost, and ptosis (lowered position) of the kidney follows. Chronic passive congestion, kinked ureters, urinary stasis, stones, and infection are possible outcomes, since the function of the kidneys is dependent on a full blood and nerve supply and on free drainage—all of which ptosis may disturb. The normal position of the kidneys can be restored and the protective fat replaced by relieving the downward pressure of poor body mechanics.

Following are the main causes of kidney ptosis:

- falling on the coccyx;
- severe physical trauma;
- losing weight too quickly;
- a state of weakness and depression;
- as a consequence of giving birth (see end of chapter);
- as a consequence of surgery;
- chronic coughing.

~Kidney People~

• Depleted deep-seated energy reserves

What is the difference between deep-seated energy and superficial energy? Suppose you have a bad cold, your nose is running, it's red and irritated from all the blowing, you have hot and cold spells that wear you out. And everybody is saying (as if to make things worse), "You don't look too great!" OK, you are tired, but a bit of rest and the right diet would put you back on your feet in no time. You've only lost some of your superficial energy. Deep-seated energy is our reserve, and it helps us overcome serious physical and emotional difficulties. Severe illness, family trouble, and depression all tap into our reserves and draw from our deeper energy source to pull us out of our difficulties. The kidneys are the organ that represents this energy, particularly the left kidney.

• A lowered strength potential

Let's make a distinction between power and energy, with an analogy to electric power. The power is the source of the energy. We all have a unique initial potential. This may seem cruel, but we do not all enjoy equal energetic capacities. To each his or her motor! Certain motors, with the same power, don't produce the same energy. When they aren't working well, the kidneys eat up a lot of energy. A person with a weak link in the kidneys will have a decreased power source. The strength potential is lower to begin with for a kidney person.

• Existential fear

Fear is ancestral and deeply rooted in us. We bear it in our genes. There is no life without fear—fear of fire, water, earthquakes, lightning, catastrophes, of being wounded, of death. This existential fear deep inside us lurks ready to jump out whenever any more or less serious danger signal appears. When someone's weak link is their kidneys, this existential fear is more firmly rooted and causes more problems.

• Reactive fear

Reactive fear is connected to a specific cause. It is powerful, intense, and closely linked to a negatively perceived event. For example, Joseph is a good driver, but one winter evening in terrible weather, an icy patch on the road gets the better of him. In a curve, he loses control of his car and slides, then falls over the retaining wall and stops just short of a ditch, with two wheels in mid-air. Feeling that the car is about to tumble into the ditch, Joseph grips the steering wheel, not daring to budge. More than an hour goes by before some people passing by stop to help. Several of them hang on to the back of the car to keep it from slipping while he gets out. The next day, Joseph has a 104°F fever and a bad urinary tract infection, the first one he's ever had. It's the after-effect of the intense fear he went through, hanging in thin air, not knowing whether he would come out alive.

• Fear of being abandoned

We are endowed with a highly developed need to be loved that shows up even from the youngest age. We need to be loved by our mother first of all, and later by loved ones in our close circles: our parents and grandparents, our lover or partner. Later on, our own children. When someone leaves us, it feels like losing a bit of ourselves. "If the other person leaves me, I lose all my bearings, I lose myself, I am lost! That is why I am so afraid." It is so much more comfortable to feel secure! When we feel abandoned, rightfully so or not, the kidneys can react by provoking an infection, stones, or high blood pressure.

• A great feeling of insecurity

Kidney people never seem to feel secure. They try to suppress the lurking fear by being overly active—for example, by working too hard to ensure their family's financial security—or on an emotional level, by taking all sorts of precautions that will weigh down a relationship. However, relationships cannot be based on fear.

• Deep-seated anger

This deep anger has nothing to do with the temporary flare-ups we express when one of our children loses the car keys we entrusted him with, or treats the precious collector's books we lent her carelessly. Like existential fear, deep-seated anger lies huddled up inside us. It rumbles like magma inside a volcano. This is demanding, frustrated anger. It sets off the sympathetic nervous system, the one that excites and stimulates us.

As a baby, Patrick used to have surprisingly intense fits of anger. Nothing would calm him down. "In those moments, it felt like he was angry with the whole world," his mother comments. Now an adult, he still has violent and irrational fits of anger. He has gone into therapy to try to get over them. Patrick is very much aware of his behavior. He says, "I have this huge, demanding power within me, it's as strong and unwillingly destructive as a tidal wave. I sometimes even feel resentful toward my parents because I am alive, but I can't explain why." The therapy helps him tame his anger a bit. But people around him have also adapted, by keeping a distance and avoiding confrontation with him. By staying clear of an angry person, we save ourselves psychological pain.

Patrick, strangely enough, does not have specific kidney trouble. But when his mother was pregnant with him, because he was not in an optimal position, she suffered three attacks of pyelonephritis (kidney infections), which she often told him about.

The first time Patrick came to see me, my fingers were constantly attracted toward his kidneys. I asked, "Do you have any kidney problems?"

"No, not that I know of," Patrick responded.

The same thing happened the second time he came, and that is when Patrick told me about his mother's kidney infections, adding, "I don't know why, but every time she would mention it, I felt responsible." Patrick had actually come to me because of lumbago that was bothering him, especially in the morning. His mother and he had several very frank discussions about the issue. These conversations, along with the Visceral Manipulation treatment, solved the problem.

• A need to surpass oneself

Do heroes have two enormous kidneys? This is just to say that kidney people sometimes manifest a need to outdo themselves, to push beyond their limits, and to commit themselves to great causes. They almost overdo it. They need to prove to themselves that they are capable of facing up to difficult challenges. Surpassing themselves is in their nature. This can go from amateur sporting performance to wild acts of courage, not to mention intellectual or spiritual quests or a Stakhanovist attitude at work. It isn't necessarily to prove their abilities to others (as we saw with stomach people)—it's for themselves. They have this strength within themselves.

Take Ghislaine, for example, who lives in the mountains. During a trip with her son, she loses control of the wheel. The car falls into a ditch full of water. Water starts seeping in and the level rises dangerously. "I thought my son was going to drown and this rage took hold of me," she explains. "I don't know where I found the strength, but I got out through the one door that was not underwater and tugged at that car to pull it out of the water." When the rescue squad arrived, they just couldn't understand how a slight little woman like her had managed to make a heavy car move. "Nothing could have stopped me," says Ghislaine. "This energy and power coming from my kidneys astounded me! Whenever I encounter a problem, I concentrate on the kidney area, and it makes me feel stronger."

• Generosity

Generosity is natural to kidney people. They will help others in all circumstances, unfailingly and spontaneously. You can also count on them to put some pep into a group, a gathering, an association—the life of the party!

• A need to lead

Full of energy and enthusiasm when their kidneys are doing well, kidney people are convinced that they are right and ardently need to convince others. They have a hard time with people contradicting them and not following their lead in implementing ideas and projects. It gives them lower back pain that is due not to vertebral problems, but to the kidneys; the pain sometimes constricts their breathing. Power of persuasion is their shield, a form of self-protection without a real reason. It's an impulsive attitude. Usually, conviction confirms leaders in their impulses and gives them the strength to act. But this doesn't mean they are self-assured. On the contrary, kidney people are often full of doubt.

• Pessimism that comes in cycles

Kidney people can be full of energy and enthusiasm, but they also go through spells of fatigue and pessimism. When their kidneys are not working as well as they should, they lose a lot of their natural pep.

"Genitality," or Our Reproductive Potential

This neologism is used by various authors and not necessarily to mean the same thing. To me, genitality is our reproductive potential as well as the origins of our own existence. Again, we are referring to a potential and not necessarily to reproduction itself. Everyone has the power to procreate. This potential will be lived out or not. Some kidney women who don't have children have a more motherly attitude toward their loved ones than do some biological mothers.

Sexual energy. The left kidney is the main partner of our feminine or masculine power. It's a potential we have within us, and (as with genitality) we make more or less use of it. Some people don't have a sexual partner but display the energy linked to sexual instinct and obvious sensuality. I remember a nun who used to come to see me for recurrent infections in her left kidney. She had a very feminine aura about her; she walked and moved with a lot of charm, and her graceful movements attracted the eye. She was aware of this but had chosen to devote herself to God, body and soul. She spoke quite openly about it: "I would have been just as loving and enthusiastic a wife if I had gotten married. This energy is in me, and I chose to devote it to God. I am genuinely happy about it." However, at some level, either the suppression of her sexual energy led to the recurring kidney infections, or the recurrent kidney infections suppressed her sexual energy.

Our biological connection with our genitors. This is every human being's fundamental relationship. Nobody can deny the connection that unites us with our genitors, whether or not we are happy about who they are or were. Some people might even be in permanent conflict with their parent(s), but an irresistible power always leads them back to them. Certain adopted children will not rest until they have reconnected with their genitors, and they put so much determination into it that they can develop kidney dysfunction.

Marie-Hélène had been an orphan on welfare. She has everything she needs to be a happy woman today—a comfortable life, two happily married children, activities she is devoted to…. And yet, she spent a fortune and fifteen years of her life trying to find her father. (She knew her mother.) When she finally found his trace, he was two years dead. But the most important thing for her was to find confirmation of her own existence and identity. She told me, "I felt instantaneous relief. Seeing a picture of him filled me with an unexplainable feeling. I don't know what to call it—maybe the feeling of filiation that had been suppressed. I had gotten this idea that I had to put a face on my father. Suddenly something let go in me, physically, especially in the kidneys. I stopped getting kidney infections."

How to Take Care of the Kidneys

From a physical point of view

- Avoid remaining seated for too long.
- Be sure to stay active, at least periodically, during long trips. If you're flying, get up at least once an hour and stretch your legs. If you're traveling by car, you should stop and walk a bit every hour or so.

Pregnancy and the Kidneys. During pregnancy, the baby sometimes compresses the mother's kidneys, causing lumbago and urinary tract infections. The pain often radiates into the thighs and even the knees. The kidneys, unlike the other organs, are not firmly attached by ligaments. They stay in place thanks to our abdominal muscle tone. During pregnancy, under the effect of hormones, this muscle tone diminishes. The considerable effort needed to push when giving birth, in addition to the decreased muscle tone, pulls the kidneys downward. The right kidney is more often affected, because it is already naturally in a lower position—beneath the liver—than the left kidney. A kidney that slides lower than its normal place will tend to become congested. It won't eliminate as well as it should and will be prone to producing crystals or stones. A practitioner can help by working on the kidneys with Visceral Manipulation, which can decongest the kidneys and help them regain better mobility. Our purpose is not to put them back in their place, but to make them more functional.

Falling on Your Backside. It happens often, and unfortunately it tends to make other people laugh, but not the person who falls. A blow to the kidney area can have serious consequences: back pain, a drop in blood pressure, ptosis (prolapse) of the bladder and uterus, headaches, etc. In the event of kidney ptosis, a properly trained manual therapy practitioner can help by working with the coccyx and spine. A manual therapist can help by working on the soft tissues associated with the coccyx and the spine, as well as applying Visceral Manipulation to the kidneys.

From a nutritional point of view

Avoid or reduce your intake of:

- Protein from animal sources, especially in the evening: red meat, cheese, milk, cold cuts, milk products (yogurt, creams, and puddings), seafood, offal (liver, kidney, tongue). A diet high in animal protein affects certain minerals in the urine that may promote the formation of kidney stones.
- Salt. You can replace it with herbs. Check the ingredients in prepared foods and beverages. The food industry tends to use a lot of salt for taste and to create an addiction. You'll find salt in places you wouldn't have suspected it: in jam, soda, ready-made dishes, etc. Reducing sodium in the diet appears to reduce the amount of calcium excreted in the urine. Consequently, people who develop stones containing calcium may benefit from a low sodium intake.
- Sparkling mineral water rich in sodium.
- Meat that is too fatty or cooked in fatty gravy.
- Too much beer. In small quantities it's a diuretic, but more than two or three beers at a time will wear out the kidneys.

Important to know:

We should all be cautious of the side effects of medicines, especially nonsteroidal anti-inflammatory drugs (NSAIDs). As the name implies, they quell pain by quieting inflammation and can be particularly hard on the kidneys, causing fibrosis and rigidity and, in extreme cases, kidney failure. Carefully read the instructions enclosed with the medicine to be informed of undesirable side effects.

Recommended:

- Drink often but only a little at a time. Body fluids contain electrolytes (particularly sodium compounds, such as sodium chloride) in concentrations that must be held within very narrow limits. Water enters the body orally and leaves the body primarily in urine, sweat, and exhaled water vapor. If water enters the body more quickly than it can be removed, body fluids are diluted and a potentially dangerous shift in electrolyte balance occurs. Beware of the theory going around about drinking two to three quarts of liquid a day. Water consumption depends upon each individual's physiological parameters—their activity level as well as heat and humidity factors. A 175-pound person does not have the same requirements as a 110-pound person. An athlete or a blue-collar worker drinks more than a person whose job is sedentary. The main thing is to drink according to your thirst, in small quantities, and preferably lukewarm. Cold liquids are emptied from the stomach at a faster rate than fluids at body temperature, so less can be absorbed.
- Forcing yourself to drink too much overburdens your kidneys. A bit of freshly squeezed grapefruit juice mixed with a lot of water, is excellent for your kidneys. Make yourself diuretic herbal teas—particularly thyme, rosemary, kidney vetch, or cherry stems. When practicing

sports or doing hard physical work, especially if it requires endurance, drink in small quantities. A person with sensitive kidneys who doesn't drink enough while doing demanding physical work might accumulate toxins or develop kidney stones. Moreover, because of sweating, the urine is very concentrated and less fluid.

- Eat such foods as leek, papaya, potatoes, spinach, endive, zucchini, apples, grapefruit. They help with bowel elimination, as well as help the kidneys to metabolize and eliminate proteins.
- Eat fiber-rich fruits and vegetables (broccoli, string beans, peas, tomato, sorrel, leek, endive). They are good for you in all circumstances. They help prevent dehydration, for one, as well as boost the immune system, neutralize free radicals, and decrease risks for cancer.

From a psychological point of view

Learn to control your fear and anger. Learn to distinguish between existential fear and the fear you experience when faced with concrete danger. The fear which is buried deep inside you can come out in the form of anger or aggressiveness. Avoid situations that might put you off balance unexpectedly, and take things step by step.

Mylène, one of my patients, has always been afraid of the dark, to the point of not daring to step out of her house after nightfall. One night she decided that she had had enough of this phobia, and she started making herself go out every night and take a few steps around her house when it was pitch-black. "At the beginning," she explains, "I couldn't even breathe, and I would run. Then, with each step, I began breathing in deeply and concentrating on the sound of my breath. This way I no longer heard the noises in the dark. Since then, I've solved the problem, and I use the same technique when I feel anger rising in me. Breathing consciously helps me relax, first the body and then the mind."

15

The Bladder:
Constant Control

The bladder is located behind the pubis and collects the urine that the kidneys produce. Water accumulates toxins on its way through the body. After being processed by the kidneys, the water pours into the bladder as urine, constantly and in small quantities. The bladder fills up little by little and stretches. Once the urine volume has reached twelve fluid ounces (a little under a pint), we feel the urge to urinate. The bladder is able to contain up to about twenty-seven fluid ounces of urine. The kidneys produce about one and a half quarts (fifty fluid ounces) of urine a day.

How the Bladder Works

The bladder can be compared to a reservoir with a valve or faucet. Like a faucet, the urethral sphincter keeps the bladder shut. That is what is called continence. We decide by an act of the will to open the "faucet" to urinate. We relax the sphincter just long enough to let the urine out. When we can't control this sphincter anymore, we begin to have what are called "incontinence problems." The valve has stretched and urine leaks out when we strain in physical effort, or maybe when we laugh or cough. Women are more prone to incontinence after difficult pregnancies, births that occurred too quickly or were induced, operations in the abdomen, or falls where they hurt their coccyx. Because a woman's pelvis is wider than a man's, the bladder has more room to move around and get in the wrong position. Similarly, the uterus, often retroversed—also known as a tipped uterus (the uterus is tipped toward the back rather than forward)—drags the bladder down toward the bottom of the pelvis.

When the Bladder Doesn't Work as well as It Should

• Incontinence

With incontinence, there is a definite feeling of no longer being able to control the bladder's sphincter sufficiently. There will be a frequent need to urinate, leaving the impression that the bladder hasn't been completely emptied. There is a feeling of weight in the lower abdomen. The most common causes are births where the tissues had a rough time, surgery, a chronic cough, physical trauma, menopause, depression, lack of physical mobility, and aging.

• Infections

A woman's urethra is five times shorter than a man's, and closer to the anus. This is what causes more frequent urinary infections (cystitis) in women. Some women also suffer from urine reflux from the bladder into the ureters (the tubes that lead from the kidneys into the bladder).

• Burning

This is usually cystitis, more often than not with no germs involved. When inflammation of the bladder is not caused by bacteria, it is known as interstitial cystitis, the cause of which is still an enigma to the medical community. This book sheds light on that mysterious cause.

• Cramps

The bladder is a muscle. Therefore it contracts, and sometimes it has a hard time letting go again. You feel a weight above the pubis.

• And what about men?

Men generally don't have the kind of incontinence problems linked to effort that women have, except in certain cases of prostate trouble or neurological dysfunction. Women have a wider pelvis, and their thighbones are set differently. This can destabilize the bladder. Pregnancies and births create mechanical tensions which affect the bladder and often pull it downward, causing incontinence. Furthermore, when a woman's intestines are tense, tight, and full of air—and because of the extra width of the hips—they can put more pressure on the bladder.

~Bladder People~

• The organ of education

It is not always easy, from an emotional standpoint, to separate the bladder from the genital organs. In women, it is easier to analyze the emotional significance of the bladder, as females from a young age typically get messages (conscious or subconscious) that they must always be clean and be concerned about smell. Also, the genital area is more difficult to clean for females than males. The bladder is also subject to educational pressure during childhood. This is particularly true of women who were raised within the old-fashioned training system, along the lines of "reward and punishment." This necessarily brings guilt and frustration in its wake. A strict education, discipline, prohibitions, and old-fashioned beliefs develop uncontrolled fears and guilt feelings in women, such as fear of their body and fear of not being clean. These tensions have an influence on the bladder and can cause inflammation as well as other problems.

In regard to the bladder, men are typically not affected in the same manner as women. The genital area for men is easy to clean. The men's area of concern (more so a weak link for men than women) relates to sexual function.

• The importance of control

The bladder being the object of almost permanent management becomes a larger symbol of control and can produce attitudes such as not being able to let go, never relaxing, never escaping control. On the street, bladder people take small steps; they feel out of place in society because they are afraid to disturb other people. Women will more often have bladder issues due to the nature of their anatomy, as well as societal judgments. Bladder women often feel guilty because as children their duties were emphasized more than their rights. They were probably taught to always be helpful and more attentive to others than to themselves. Moreover, in some cases, women were also taught a whole series of taboos, such as "pleasures of the body are to be considered suspicious" or "sexuality is to be condemned." This kind of education produces "good wives" who are submissive toward their husbands, but are often dissatisfied and inhibited women who harbor unresolved guilt feelings and suppress their true sentiments. Bladder women are also reserved, discreet, shy, often submissive. They have a hard time making decisions and expressing themselves.

• Emotional blackmail and guilt

During the toilet-training period, parents often exert unconscious emotional blackmail on their toddlers, whether girls or boys, roughly along these lines: "If you use the potty, you're nice to Mommy and Daddy," "If you don't use the potty, you're not nice to them." And at that age, it is so important to make your parents happy, not angry! Reiterated emotional blackmail of this kind can cause problems in a child's urinary and psychological behavior. Guilt is the logical consequence of emotional blackmail. At an age where becoming toilet-trained is a difficult skill to acquire and throughout the training period, the child will automatically feel guilty if his or her parents aren't satisfied. These constantly reinforced guilt feelings will reappear later, when the child has grown up.

One of my patients, Sylvie, has two children who apparently haven't attained the social success that she hoped they would. "I did everything I could," she says, "but I know it's my fault. It's not their fault." As a reflection of her children's social and professional tribulations, Sylvie gets recurrent bladder infections. Strangely enough, no medical test has shown any physical cause or any trace of infection. The cystitis is directly triggered by Sylvie's worry over her children.

• Obedience and submission

It is often said that rules are made to be broken! But challenge is not everyone's cup of tea. Some people prefer to avoid confrontation. They are submissive toward anyone who makes a show of authority: their father, their boss, their husband, a friend. Bladder people can't stand tension and will do anything they can to avoid it.

• Prudishness

Prudishness is often due to educational or relationship pressure. Children have no particular prudishness in them until puberty, an age where body consciousness becomes all-important. Teenagers cover their body, lock the bathroom door, ask their mother not to take them all the way to school, not to give them a kiss in front of their friends.... It is a time when the body is changing, and with it, the adolescent's view of society and family. Teenagers lose the landmarks they had, in their body and relationships. If they were fed guilt-producing messages during childhood, this can have disastrous consequences. Even when the teenager has succeeded in accepting his or her own body, he or she still has to accept other people's bodies for what they are.

• Cyclical shyness

Some people are shy by nature, in all circumstances. Bladder people (those with a weakness in the bladder area) have shy episodes, depending on the feedback they get, but also based on their physical state. A patient comes to see me for recurrent back pain that doesn't seem to have a mechanical cause. The lower part of her abdomen shows very great muscular tension. I ask, "Why are you so tense in that part of your body? Do you have pelvic pain?" (To get people to be more open about their incontinence problems, it is often better to speak of abdominal pain to open the discussion.)

She responds, "No, no pain, but I sometimes have a little leakage, and I tighten my muscles to prevent it." Then my patient confides, "When I have incontinence problems, I feel like hiding in a rat hole. I feel myself withdrawing, and I don't dare look anyone in the eye. I feel ashamed. Yes, that's it, I'm ashamed."

After a few sessions of Visceral Manipulation on her bladder and osteopathic manipulation to her lumbar area, the problems disappear: "I've regained confidence and joy," she says, looking me straight in the eye.

Today people speak more freely about this subject, which has become less of a taboo. They know that re-education, Visceral Manipulation, manual therapy, and in extreme cases surgery can free them quickly from the discomforts of those leaks.

How to Take Care of the Bladder

From a physical point of view

- It is important to have a strong, mobile, and supple spine. All the nerves in the bladder come from the vertebrae, the sacrum, and the coccyx. Falls on your coccyx can have unforeseeable consequences: don't wait to go see an osteopath or manual therapist.
- Any surgery in the abdomen will leave you with adhesions which can affect the bladder. Visceral Manipulation, massage and physical therapy, osteopathy, and exercise can free you from these adhesions.
- Excess weight, especially in the abdomen, deprives the bladder of adequate mobility and pushes it downward.
- Make sure your feet are solidly rooted on the ground. I have seen patients suffer from incontinence following a trauma to their legs or feet (sprains, breaks). When you're not walking comfortably, mechanical factors can set the bladder off balance.

From a nutritional point of view

- The main thing is to drink often and a little at a time. Excess water in the bladder increases tension in its walls and causes inner pressure. Make sure you empty your bladder: keeping it full will make its muscles thicken and will also increase inner pressure.
- Drink low-sodium water.
- Reduce your intake of dietary bladder irritants: alcoholic beverages, carbonated beverages (with or without

caffeine), milk or milk products, coffee or tea (even decaffeinated), medicines with caffeine, salt, red meat, seafood, high-acid citrus fruits and juices, tomatoes and tomato-based products, highly spiced/hot foods, sugar, honey, chocolate, corn syrup, artificial sweetener.

• Watch out for constipation—it is the bladder's enemy. The lower part of the intestine which leans on the bladder can increase its pressure and push the bladder downward.

• Surgery in the abdomen will leave you with adhesions that can affect the bladder. Systemic enzymes can help your body break down the internal and external adhesions.

From a psychological point of view

• Try therapies that will help you gain self-confidence and fight your shyness and fear of facing others. Apart from psychotherapy, singing and dancing are excellent activities to promote confidence and muscle tone. Standing up straight is the most fundamental therapy. Walk with an upright gait, keeping your shoulders back. Practice at home first and then outdoors, looking people in the eye.

• Free yourself from that "reward-punishment" system, the strictness, or simply the message you received from your parents: "Be a good girl or boy—you have to go on the potty to make Mommy and Daddy happy." This message heaps guilt upon bladder people, who feel that they always have to be helpful and in their best mood. In constant fear of other people's judgment, bladder people have to work on not feeling responsible for everything, on allowing themselves an occasional bad mood, and on no longer playing the role of a little kid still under the parents' thumb.

16

The Genital Organs:
Our Origin and Future

The genital organs (vagina, uterus, ovaries, fallopian tubes, prostate, penis, testicles, breasts) constitute the human sexual and reproductive system. It is a highly elaborate system, which differentiates men from women and sets up the meeting of these two complementary beings for the continuity of the human race. What is so beautiful about this reciprocal male/female mechanism is that procreation can be the result of pleasure and the merging of two beings, expressing their shared love and joy.

How the Genitals Work

The genital system is dependent upon the hormones secreted by the brain and the suprarenal glands (tiny glands located just above the kidneys, also known as the adrenal glands). Hormonal stimulation, sometimes measured in thousandths of billionths of grams, takes place within a very subtle environment. This is what you might call extreme precision!

If we look at the emotional significance of the genitalia in women, aside from the breasts, it is difficult to distinguish among the different genital organs' influence. The uterus and the ovaries seem to react to the same psychological factors. Certain types of stress can have a sudden effect on the pituitary gland's hormonal production and cause immediate vaginal bleeding. In general, disturbances in the genital area are set off by the brain. But there can be local causes: gynecological problems linked to giving birth, to surgery, infections, falls, or spinal and coccyx problems. In men, the prostate is definitely the most vulnerable genital organ.

Women, or Yin

In Chinese medicine and philosophy, yin is the cosmic feminine element and yang the masculine one. To a certain extent, yin represents passivity, whereas yang is movement. But yin and yang are inseparable. This duality can be found in our physiological makeup. Commanded by the brain, the woman's ovaries produce estrogens, progesterone (yin), and a small quantity of testosterone (yang). These hormones determine women's morphological characteristics: the breadth of the pelvis, developed breasts, the thickness and texture of the skin, pubic hair, etc.

Estrogens. Produced by the ovaries, estrogens are hormones derived from cholesterol. The suprarenal glands and the placenta also produce estrogens in small quantities. The liver eliminates estrogens in the form of cholesterol, which in turn can intoxicate the liver. Paradoxically, estrogens reduce the cholesterol level. It may be a result of this active estrogen production that women rarely suffer from coronary disease before menopause. On the other hand, estrogens increase the bile's viscosity and slow down its excretion. This makes women more susceptible to gallbladder stones, especially during the second part of their cycle, between the fourteenth and the twenty-eighth day. A drop in the level of estrogens (such as during menopause) also play a major role in the development of osteoporosis.

Progesterone. Produced mainly by the ovaries and to a certain extent by the placenta, this hormone prepares the woman's body to give birth each month. It contributes to the development of the uterus and the breasts. Among other things, it plays an essential role during pregnancy by helping to dilate the blood vessels, which ensures better nurturing of the fetus. The regularly shifting balance of estrogen and progesterone is vital to many aspects of a woman's health, whether she is pregnant or not, or even fertile or not.

The ovum. All women are born with a store of approximately two million ova, which reside in the two ovaries. They will not produce any more. By puberty, they have only about 400,000 left, the rest having died and been eliminated from the body. The ova remain inactive from birth until puberty and can play their role in procreation from puberty to menopause. About 400,000 ova: that may seem like a lot, but it's not much compared to the 80 million sperm usually present in a single ejaculation. The ova mature in the course of the twenty-eight-day ovarian cycle (when everything is working properly). Ovulation takes place on the fourteenth day. Only one ovary is involved in each ovulation: the two ovaries take turns. One day before ovulation, body temperature increases about 3 degrees Fahrenheit until the period begins. Some women—if their cycle was predictably regular—have used this phenomenon as a contraceptive method (the Ogino method). It's far from being one hundred percent reliable! Some people were born thanks to this method.

The uterus: the embryo's nest. The uterus is the baby's shelter. It is where the embryo is protected, kept warm, and fed. From an emotional point of view, this notion of a shelter is essential. The uterus is also a powerful muscle, able to expel the fetus once it has reached its term. The cervix secretes a mucus that keeps exterior germs from reaching the fetus. It also secretes cervical mucus, which is more viscous and alkaline during ovulation, to help the sperm make their way to the ovum.

Men, or Yang

In men, the hormonal mechanisms are much less complex than in women. The testicles—tiny sperm factories—also produce testosterone and very small quantities of estrogen. (Don't forget that there is some yin in men and some yang in women.) But today men are producing less and less sperm, for reasons that are hard to prove: factors that have been implicated include tight pants, which increase the temperature in the testicles, pollution in the air and in food, stress, and possibly estrogen-like substances in hormone-fed meats and the plastic bottles and wrappers which leach into food items. The scrota containing the testicles are separate little compartments that are usually able to protect the sperm from the harmful effects of too high a temperature. You could say that they are two insulated bags which bring the temperature inside the testicles down several degrees lower than the outdoor temperature. They adapt to changes in weather. When it is hot outside, the scrota stretch to move the testicles further away from the warm body, and when it is cold, they shorten. Kept at the right temperature, sperm are very active. Sperm have a life span of two to five days and secrete prostaglandin which stimulates the opening of the cervix as well as contractions of the uterus and the fallopian tubes. All this helps the sperm along their way to the ovum.

The male hormone: testosterone. In both sexes, the suprarenal glands produce small quantities of testosterone, which (like estrogens in women) is derived from cholesterol. Testosterone gives men their morphological characteristics: shoulders wider than the pelvis, more body hair on the limbs and torso, more developed muscles than in women, sebaceous glands that function differently. It also has an effect on behavior. If you watch young children playing outdoors, you'll notice, of course, that the girls and the boys play very different games: to paint a rather broad and generalized picture, the boys will be fighting and the girls playing house or hopscotch or something else cooperative!

Testosterone manages the libido (sexual desire), which is said to make men's heads spin, and to which we add emotion, of course! We need cholesterol to produce this hormone: at one point, doctors were working so hard on reducing their patients' cholesterol level that some men suffered from hormone and immune deficiency.

The prostate. This small chestnut-shaped gland encircles the urethra, the canal that leads from the bladder to the penis. It is found only in men. About thirty percent of the liquid in an ejaculation is made up of prostate secretions. They reduce the acidity level in the vagina (sperm do not like acidity) and make the cervix more flexible, facilitating penetration. The secretions also contain sugar (fructose) which gives the sperm strength for their perilous trip into the fallopian tubes, and enzymes which increase their speed. Only about two thousand sperm will be strong enough to reach the uterus and the fallopian tubes. In order for fertilization to occur, one of these sperm must attach itself to the ovum and penetrate its outer surface. The fertilized ovum will then continue travelling down the fallopian tube, taking several days until it reaches the uterus. When it arrives, it attaches to the lining of the uterus and continues to grow.

The Importance of Our Sense of Smell

Like other animals, we secrete minute quantities of chemical substances known as pheromones, which are capable of arousing physical attraction in members of our species. A natural phenomenon—one of the subtleties of creation! Did you know that a male butterfly can sense a female more than six miles away? An impressive performance, knowing the area that a butterfly takes up in space! Anyone who has a dog knows that a male dog will smell a female in heat from miles away. I address this olfactory sense in this chapter on the genitals because of its obvious importance in attraction and procreation, the major function of the genitals.

Bees, whose highly organized social behavior has been the subject of numerous studies, produce different kinds of pheromones which help regulate life in the hive.*

For example, the queen bee produces pheromones that will block the female bees' ovarian cycle at certain times, so they can concentrate entirely on their work in the hive. These famed pheromones have an effect on the bees' neuronal and metabolic development. The nurse bees, who usually start gathering pollen at the age of three weeks, can be "programmed" by the pheromones produced by the queen bee, to begin this function much earlier, if necessary for the hive. Humans function along similar instinctive lines, although most of us are not acutely conscious of this.

In humans pheromones are mainly secreted by the sebaceous glands connected to the hair, the underarms, and the genital organs. They let off a subtle odor, which can hardly be quantified. Let's take the example of garlic for a benchmark: its distinctive smell can be perceived when the concentration is around ten-billionths of a gram per cubic meter of air. So as you can see, our perception of smells must be quite subtle to be able to capture the scent of pheromones, whose concentration is infinitesimal. There is a long tradition among perfume-makers of mixing musk and other animal hormones with floral or spicy scents to make sure that perfumes play their seductive role.

---

* Isabelle Leoncini and Yves le Conte studied these different functions at the Laboratory for Biology and the Protection of Bees at the National Institute of Agronomic Research, France.

Alert Senses

When we come close to someone, our first relationship is not verbal, but visual and instinctive. Even before we shake hands and say hello, we perceive sensorial information:

- With our eyes, we grasp a face, an attitude, gestures.
- With what we could call our "intuition," we sense the other person's electromagnetic field. You can visualize it as a halo (the person's warmth or the aura they give off) emanating from every living being. It is a very real thing and can be photographed with special equipment. Some people speak of an aura which combines physical and psychological radiance.
- With our sense of smell, we gain information about the other person. Smell is one of the first senses that primitive humans developed when perfecting their survival instinct. They knew how to detect the presence of an enemy (or the scent of a woman) quite precisely, and at a distance. The smell coming from a woman's hair is not the same before and after her period: this proves that hormonal changes affect the odor we give off. Studies have shown that women who live in a community situation often have their period at the same time. The pheromones produced by a few women just before menstruation apparently stimulate the pituitary gland and hypothalamus of the entire group and set off simultaneous periods.

When we can't gain information from our sense of smell, or can't seem to figure a person out, we instinctively know that we are missing something. There is a common expression in French—*"Je ne sais pas pourquoi mais je ne peux pas le sentir!"*—meaning "I don't know why, but I can't 'smell' that person!" In other words, "I can't figure him out, what his motives are, who he really is," etc. This everyday French idiom describes instinctive and often unexplainable feelings. It is hard to prove anything in this field of study. We are dealing with molecules of the order of billionths of grams, but many people think (or sense!) that smells play an important role in our way of approaching, appreciating, and getting to know other people.

When the Genitals Don't Work as well as They Should

The genital organs are the core of our potential for fertility and maternity/paternity, of physical attraction, of impulses, of love games, of sexual satisfaction, and of physical pleasure.

In Men

The male genital system may send the following messages when it is out of balance:

- An unpleasant feeling in the lower abdomen.
- A frequent need to urinate.
- Difficulties in urinating (less powerful flow, insufficiently emptied bladder).
- Difficulties ejaculating.
- Inefficient erections.
- A decrease in libido.

In men's subconscious and conscious mind, the fear of not being sexually "up to par" is all-powerful. It often takes a long time for them to understand that sex is not an endurance contest. Nonetheless, partial or definitive impotence can have disastrous effects on a man's psyche. The prostate is very hormone-dependent and reacts very strongly to any imbalance (hormonal or otherwise). It can enlarge and compress the urethra, making men have to get up at night to urinate. The need to empty their bladder can become pressing, and ejaculation can become more and more labored.

In Women

When the female reproductive system is not functioning at its peak, one or more of the following symptoms may be present as a message:

- Painful, irregular, or absent periods.
- Unusual local odors.
- Vaginal discharge or bleeding.
- Ovarian cysts.
- Uterine fibroids.
- Heaviness and pain in the lower abdomen and in the legs.
- Lumbago.
- Painful or unsatisfying sexual relations.
- A lack of libido.
- Infertility.

The female genital system is incomparably more complex than the male system. Women's hormonal system affects their entire organism to a much more obvious degree than do the male hormones in men. Premenstrual syndrome is one of the best illustrations of this fact: a bloated abdomen, increase in weight, congestion or sensitivity in the breasts, headaches, nausea, acceleration of the heartbeat, pre-depressive states, hypersensitivity, hot and cold flushes, and more can all beset the woman whose hormones have gone awry for a few days. A healthy hormonal balance in women can eliminate many of these symptoms.

Menopause. This is one of the main natural stages in a woman's life, as is puberty in youth. Painless in some women and a real struggle for others, menopause is the cause of many changes in the body, and other variable symptoms:

- When a woman fails to stay physically fit in middle age, her waistline will tend to widen and her ribs will sag toward the pelvis, causing a loss of muscle tone in the abdomen.
- Many women tend to gain weight more easily at this stage of life, in part because hormones have a direct impact on appetite, metabolism, and fat storage. Also, women at mid-life typically exercise less, eat more, and burn fewer calories.
- Some women experience a sagging of the tissues that hold up the bladder and the uterus (prolapse).

- The breasts change: the decrease in hormone levels depletes the breast tissues, but their fat content, which makes up 95% of the breast volume, increases.
- Menopause can also bring in its wake hot flashes, insomnia, nausea, vaginal dryness, and circulatory problems.

Not easy to accept, along with entering the fateful fifties! But there's no need to panic: the picture we've just painted sums up all the inconveniences that can go along with menopause, and you will probably only experience a few, if any, of the symptoms. Maintain good health and fitness, and you will find menopause much easier.

Headaches. Some women get headaches at regular points in their ovarian cycle. Medicine is still largely at a loss when it comes to helping alleviate hormone-related headaches. With the onset of menopause, the fall in estrogen and progesterone levels tends to make the headaches disappear. The other side of the coin is that cholesterol and triglyceride levels increase with menopause. Of all the hormone-related headaches, the most difficult to treat are the kind that disappear during pregnancy and then come back again.

Hormone replacement therapy. It is hard to find the truth in the controversy over whether hormone replacement therapy (HRT) is a risk factor or a relief. American and British findings, which are contested in French medical circles, have emphasized certain dangers, particularly an increase in breast cancer risk. It would also appear that HRT's influence on preventing osteoporosis is negligible. Today gynecologists are becoming less and less keen on prescribing hormones systematically, beginning to reserve this treatment mainly for women who suffer serious problems at menopause. Bear in mind that natural treatment is always preferable to chemical solutions, which usually affects the liver and kidneys because they must detoxify the body of the excess foreign hormones. Furthermore, every woman reacts differently. There's no telling what might happen over the long term. There is a great deal of information available about natural treatments to decrease menopausal symptoms—you can find it in books, on the Internet, and by consulting natural healthcare professionals such as manual therapists, acupuncturists, naturopaths, and osteopaths.

A Turning Point in One's Life

Around the age of fifty is when many people finally commit to living according to their true personality. Life, now more than half over, takes on a new meaning, and our awareness of our wishes, choices, and options grows. Men are often chided for odd behavior at this time and labeled as having a "mid-life crisis," which in many cases is very real. This is a turning point in both men and women's lives. Even more than two decades ago, it appears that people today want to retain youthfulness and vitality. They don't see the need to slow down at mid-life. Just the opposite: many have the money, inclination, and time to focus on their desires. And those desires may not fit with some people's image of a person over the age of fifty.

Although some of the best years of life lie ahead, some women (particularly when they are going through menopause) and some men feel that their fifties are a time when they lose their motivation. An opening or a promotion in their career seems less attainable. They feel they cannot evolve along the social scale anymore. They feel stuck and doubt their ability to try out new activities. The children have grown up and are leaving the nest. Women do their best to be useful at all times. That is why they often go straight from being mothers to being grandmothers. They experience a lack of strength and of affection. Their marriage might, out of the power of habit, be turning from passion to attachment. And the children are no longer there to fill the gap. A woman around fifty who is single or childless can begin to feel a kind of guilt, a feeling of not having totally fulfilled her function. She might feel nostalgic, discouraged, and plagued with loneliness. There is an intense feeling of emotional emptiness. She will often lose self-confidence and not know what to do with her life. But, let me repeat this, do not get discouraged when reading this extensive list of possible difficulties. For many women, everything goes fine! It is important to emphasize this.

Andropause (Male Menopause)

Andropause is a term which refers to the time where a man's production of testosterone falls. It doesn't include as many obvious physical symptoms as does menopause in women. What may happen, though, is that sexual desire will diminish, become less frequent, and harder to fulfill. Andropause does have psychological repercussions because it often coincides with a period of professional and social upheaval. Men feel deeply and personally affected in their image as "a man." They may react with an exaggerated desire to remain young, by being overly active and seductive. They need to feel reassured and "still be in the race." Determined to keep what they have acquired, they have a hard time letting go and often come out of this period less at peace with themselves than do women of the same age.

"Retirement Age"

This expression is always loaded with meaning. Men who haven't prepared adequately for this transition feel as if they have suddenly turned into outcasts, stripped of all their power to act and exert influence. Retirement is a little bit like a military retreat—for some, it feels like defeat. We have to beat a retreat! There are no more victories in sight, only deep frustration, so difficult to express. The retired warrior goes home, and he can end up shutting himself in there. At the beginning he enjoys his well-earned rest, but little by little, insidiously, he feels something is missing—no one there anymore to pass on work to be done, to ask him for advice, or even to order him around. At the same time, he realizes that at home everything functions without his help! While he was absorbed in his career, his wife has gotten all the domestic affairs under control: no point trying to play boss in the household, educational counselor with the kids, or refrigerator manager! No one has been waiting for him to do the job. He has to learn to live with his wife, who more often than not is uncomfortable with his constant presence and has a hard time accepting it—she had become used to her independence and space. Feeling deprived of recognition, he will often feel lonely and degraded. He is unhappy and irritable. This period is a hard turn to negotiate and will have a different emotional impact on different individuals. A man who loses his job in what he feels are unjustified circumstances might feel sort of the same way.

~Genital People~

Genital-type men and women often feel the same needs, the same fears, the same emptiness, although there are certain peculiarities.

• *The need for a shelter, a cocoon*

We all have a need for protection, both for ourselves and our loved ones. It is important for us to create our own family refuge, like an animal in its den. Our house or apartment provides us with a physical shelter, but more importantly, it helps us create the family atmosphere we crave. Genital people are particularly sensitive to this. It's never much of a pleasure for them to go home to an empty house. Any living being will reassure us: if it's not a human being, it can be a dog or a cat. To feel the presence of a familiar being is essential.

• *The need to shelter others*

People who need to be sheltered and protected also need to provide shelter for others. This attitude is deeply rooted in the subconscious mind. Jacques left his family home for reasons he keeps to himself. But he can't help wanting to know what is going on in his "ex-home."

"Even if I'm no longer there, I want to go on managing my family," he explains. This situation stressed him out so badly that he developed an inflammation of the urethra and prostate, with no physiological explanation. The inflammation goes away as soon as he decided to go back home.

For a move to be well accepted, the family has to be united. A move isn't as stressful if the family members are all happy about it. If there has been a breakup in the family, death of a loved one, or a child leaving home, it's more difficult to deal with the separation.

• *The need to receive and to give*

This need is particularly prevalent in genital people. They do not like to think that they give in order to receive in return, but this is often the case.

This is also true in matters of the heart: giving love to other people to get love in return (among other things).

• Fear of being abandoned

Since genital people need to shelter and be sheltered, they have a basic fear of being abandoned. This fear, which is also characteristic of the intestines, will affect one or the other organ, depending on the person and his or her weak link.

• Fear of not doing well and of being judged

While this character trait is not a "privilege" of genital people, it is stronger in them. Being judged negatively means no longer being accepted by others, no longer feeling protected. Genital people tend to think, "If I don't perform well, or if I do something other people don't like, I'll no longer be loved, and I'll be left all alone." The very idea is unbearable to them. When they feel vulnerable, they will be defenseless and lack resources. This can manifest in women through irregular periods, distension in the lower abdomen, uterine spasms, and backaches. Men can experience lumbago, lower abdominal pain, and other imbalances to their genital system.

Traits of Genital Women

The need for motherhood. It is not always easy for a woman to accept infertility or menopause, which puts an end to her potential to give birth. Certain women in their fifties, as we have already mentioned, put all their hopes and desires into becoming grandmothers. Fibroids can be a way of expressing this loss of maternity. They can represent the child that the woman can no longer bear, or must not bear.

Fear of cutting the umbilical cord. There is no denying the deep and unique connection between a mother and her children. Unlike the father, she bears the child. This usually creates an exceptional symbiotic link, and consequently, a fear of cutting the cord later.

Jeanne is single and has no children. Over time, she transferred to her nephew her need to give motherly love to someone. She sees him often and knows everything about his life. Strangely enough, three months after her nephew marries, Jeanne finds out that she has a benign breast tumor. Worse yet, when he decides to emmigrate to Australia, she develops a tumor in her uterus. Jeanne seemed to have so forcibly projected this "motherly" relationship and its frustrations upon her nephew that it was as if they had a natural mother-son attachment.

The need to sacrifice oneself for a mission. Bénédicte has five children, which is a demanding situation and less typical today than in the past. She works all day long, earning great admiration from everyone around her. "She is so brave," people say. "She never complains...." She makes most of her children's clothes herself. Up at dawn, late to bed, she does all the family and household tasks like a perfect homebody. It is essential to her to enjoy recognition for all her multiple activities, and Bénédicte is already terrified when she thinks of the day her children will leave home. "I hope I'll become a grandmother very soon," she repeats, trying to cheer herself up. Bénédicte suffers from an early onset of menopause: hot flushes, changing moods and a depressive tendency, rashes, and red patches on her face. Genital women need to get recognition and set up difficult missions for themselves. But menopause has begun—Bénédicte can no longer have children, and her uterus reacts by producing a large fibroid.

Traits of Genital Men

Fear of losing their social position. Men need to feel highly regarded, if not indispensable. Social position and relationships within their work sphere are more important to men than to women. (But let's not forget that there can be yin in yang, and yang in yin.) When retirement is around the corner for a man, or when younger men lose their job, they feel an intense fear of falling off their pedestal. They need to keep asking themselves, "Am I still useful to society?" A great majority of men feel this way. Because the prostate becomes the weak link at andropause (and even more so for "genital men"), it reacts to the different conflicts which arise when a man reaches his fifties.

The need to be the leader. A "macho" doesn't just disappear into thin air! This kind of man is still the "leader," but a leader who is beginning to have slight genital and bladder problems. He'll often want to find purely physical explanations for certain "decreases in performance" (as he'll word it himself); he might put all the blame on his prostate. First he'll speak of his urinary problems, and he might then discreetly broach the subject of sexual dysfunction: weaker and shorter erections, difficulties ejaculating, a decrease in libido. So much prudery! Because unlike women, who see their gynecologist regularly, men are not used to discussing such matters, and they feel inadequate when the slightest sexual weakness appears.

Not seeing any future for themselves. We all know that true wisdom is to live in the present, with strength and awareness. We can't undo the past, and we don't know what the future holds, so the only stable value is the present. Genital men are afraid of a future they know they can no longer control. Their stomach may also react to these uncertainties.

What to do for the rest of one's life? Most men have put their entire life into their work. To cross the line into retirement, become idle, leave one's job or give up a passion is extremely difficult. Etienne is employed by the local town hall. He says so himself: "It's not a very prestigious job." But he is also the conductor of the town band and puts his entire soul into this hobby. He can't count the hours he's spent at parades, concerts, and rehearsals. He gives all his free time to the band, which has caused some family problems along the way, but the people in his town like him. Etienne has status.

One day, the mayor and his new team decide to put someone else in charge of the band. They tell Etienne without beating around the bush, adding, "You'll always be welcome in the band." A few weeks later, Etienne comes to see me because of lumbago, lower abdominal pain, and pain in his left leg. "I need to go to the toilet all the time—I have to get up several times a night." A scan reveals benign hypertrophy of the prostate, a logical consequence of the loss he experienced.

Fear of expressing things. Everything mentioned above (fear of no longer feeling important, the need to be the leader, seeing no future, wondering what to do with the rest of one's life) is rarely clearly stated by genital men. They are inhibited by notions such as "a man has to be strong," and "a man shouldn't complain." Instead of confiding and sharing, they withdraw. All these unspoken and suppressed tensions end up overwhelming them and attacking their body viciously, particularly in the genital area, as described above, affecting the sexual and psychological realms. Feeling devalued, such men gradually close off. That is where one of the major differences between men and women lies: women dare face up to their problems, using plain language. Men are incredibly prudish: "By the way … you know what I mean … things aren't going as well…." It takes a lot of perseverance to get them to speak their mind.

A need to draw attention to themselves. When they begin to feel useless, men can react in two opposite manners: either they become reclusive, or they try to attract attention, sometimes in an irrational and exaggerated way. In the second case, they set up unreasonable challenges for themselves. There are innumerable examples of daredevils in their sixties. Some will choose to ski down a dangerous slope to prove to everybody that they are still in great shape. Others will make an acrobatic swivel during a soccer game with "the guys." Yet other men yet will embark upon risky business ventures or financial deals.

How to Take Care of the Genitals

From a physical point of view

Women

- Practice gymnastics, water aerobics, stretching, walking, cross-country skiing, racket sports, bicycling.
- Have regular gynecological exams.
- See a properly trained manual therapy practitioner who practices Visceral Manipulation. A woman's pelvis often develops adhesions, due to births and gynecological surgery. An osteopath or manual therapist can free these adhesions and increase a woman's chances of becoming pregnant if there is a fertility problem.

Something to be aware of

Here is an astonishing example of the extreme complexity of creation: following natural catastrophes and mass-fatality accidents, more girls are born than boys. This phenomenon was verified after the 1995 earthquake in Kobe, Japan, and the 1976 explosion of the Seveso factory in Italy. It appears that stress makes Y-chromosome-carrying sperm less mobile.

Retroversion of the uterus (when the uterus is tipped toward the back rather than forward) is a frequent problem. Whenever a woman performs any physical activity, her uterus is in motion. Over the long term, a tipped uterus will naturally tend to snuggle up in the back of the pelvis, leaning on the sacrum. Retroversion causes lymph and vein problems which particularly affect the legs. Retroversion of the uterus can also trigger lumbago and sciatica. Therapists performing Visceral Manipulation can help, not by putting the uterus back in its original position, but by making it more mobile, more flexible, and less congested.

Men

- Exercise regularly—remain physically active. Stretching, particularly of the lumbar area, the pelvis, and the legs, is most important.
- Be careful with tobacco and alcohol—use sparingly or not at all. Drink water, in small quantities, but regularly.
- Any man aged fifty to sixty who feels forewarning signals of prostate hypertrophy should see a manual therapist who can perform Visceral Manipulation (after going to a doctor for a complete check-up). The practitioner can help decongest the prostate and give it more flexibility (through rectal manipulation). This treatment, when it works, can spare you surgery, which can have undesirable consequences such as retrograde ejaculation (the sperm goes into the bladder), impotence, and incontinence, to

varying degrees. As we have seen, the prostate surrounds the urethra like a ring. With age it can become enlarged and constrict the urethra. By mobilizing the prostate, the manual therapist can help relax the pressure on the urethra. These techniques are safe and efficient.

For Men and Women

Walking, swimming, bicycling, water aerobics, and gymnastics are excellent. Some studies conclude that the more senior citizens walk or remain active, the less chance they have of developing Alzheimer's, and the better equipped they are to defend themselves against other illnesses. Walking stimulates the lymphatic and venous systems of the pelvis and legs, which is excellent for the entire body. As we saw in the chapter on the brain, these activities increase cerebral circulation and help feed our billions of neurons more efficiently. This has a positive influence on our emotional and hormonal systems.

From a nutritional point of view

Women

- Certain plants (such as soy) and certain fruits (particularly citrus) contain active substances which have the same positive effects as hormones, especially estrogens. There is controversy regarding the benefits of soy versus too much phyto-estrogen from soy. Including cruciferous vegetables in your diet (such as broccoli, kale, bok choy, and sauerkraut) will help to balance out excess phyto-estrogen in your body.
- Get into the habit of drinking soy milk or eating tofu and soy yogurt, twice a week.
- Try trace elements and homeopathy. There are numerous sources of information (books or practitioners).

Men

- Eat broccoli, pumpkin seeds, and pumpkin seed oil to reduce congestion in the lower pelvic area and bring better blood and lymph circulation to your genital system.
- Take selenium and zinc (oysters, for instance, contain a lot of both).

Both

Eat foods rich in vitamin E, an antioxidant that interacts with insulin and with the sexual hormones. A deficiency can make it difficult for an ovum to settle in the uterus, among other things. It is mainly present in wheat germ, soy oil, peanuts, corn, chocolate, avocado, walnuts, and hazelnuts.

From a psychological point of view

Women

Pay a little more attention to the woman and a little less to the mother in you. Take care of yourself, your body, your personal and intellectual growth. Take up all those activities you never found time for: music, dance, going on trips with friends, surfing on the Web. If you feel judged, or especially if you fear other people's opinion, take a good look at the person who is being judgmental: what does she have that you don't have? Is it any of her business? What right does she have over you? Boost your self-confidence! You'll see that, little by little, you will start feeling less and less vulnerable.

Men

Retirement needs preparation. You shouldn't say, "I'll take care of it when the time comes."

It is important to plan new activities that will mean more to you than just "passing time." It's true that sports are indispensable, but sports alone are not enough. First of all, your know-how can be profitable to other people. Share it with organizations, with younger people. Before retiring, it's a good idea to contact friends, to plan activities and trips with them, to get involved in local management in your neighborhood or city. Great humanitarian causes need devoted people with time on their hands. This isn't true only of far-off countries—sometimes people in need are right at your doorstep. From an ecological point of view, our planet needs everyone's help. Retired people have the great advantage of having time at their disposal.

Both Men and Women

The home must remain the entire family's shelter, which everybody is happy to come back to. Prevent conflict, reduce tensions, let everyone have his or her place in the family unit. This way the house will be radiant with the personality of every member, young and old. We often underestimate the importance of our living quarters. Some houses are more welcoming than others, thanks to small details: lighting, how the furniture is arranged, the colors of the walls.... Make your home a warm and welcoming place, and you will benefit from its positive aura.

17

The Skin:
Our Showcase

Physiologists consider it a major organ: sixteen percent of the body weight and a surface of sixteen to twenty-two square feet. The skin is related to all the bodily functions. Its entire surface is irrigated and innerved, which makes it an ultra-sensitive information sensor. It is directly connected to the brain and spontaneously very reactive: "That gave me goose-bumps," "I've got him under my skin," "She really touched me." We turn pink with pleasure, red with shame, white with fear. The language of the skin uses colors.

Skin is a receptor of pleasure but also of pain, and it contacts the brain immediately to make use of speech and shout "ouch" or "ah" or "wow." Not only is our entire body wrapped in skin, but inside the body there is skin around every one of your muscles and organs. This is called "fascia." Many therapists believe that the fasciae memorize our emotions!

How the Skin Works

Suppleness, elasticity, and resistance are this organ's main histological characteristics (structure, composition, and function). The skin's thickness varies in different parts of our body, but it has the same three-layered structure everywhere: the epidermis or outer layer, the dermis which is rich in collagen and elastic fibers, and the hypodermis, the deepest layer which contains, among other things, the adipose cells.

• It protects us from aggressive elements

Like a shield, the skin provides us with a mechanical barrier against physical intrusions. Thanks to its padding, it can cushion shock, help us resist blows, and allow us to fall without breaking. Of course, when too violently attacked, the skin tears and can no longer offer our bones and organs sufficient protection. But it is very resistant. The skin is also an immune barrier, capable of warding off "invaders" in the form of those billions of viruses and bacteria that lurk in our environment. It defends us against chemical agents and UV radiation as well.

• It absorbs and exchanges

The skin shields us, but it also absorbs. An amazing exchange takes place at all times through our skin. Certain hormone replacement treatments are given via a patch on the skin. I remember a physical therapist who ended up with an ulcer because he used anti-inflammatory cream all day long when giving massages. His hands were so highly impregnated that the undesirable side effects of anti-inflammatory medicine crossed the barrier of his skin. A rare but telling case!

• It balances the water in our body

It is vital for us to preserve the water that makes up the largest part of our body. Every day we store and lose water (urine, sweat)—about 2.5 quarts (85 fluid ounces) gained and the same amount lost for a 155-pound man. When you sit in a bathtub, you may notice how soon you need to urinate. Water is absorbed through the skin, and to keep the vital level of water in the body, you will need to expel the excess after a while.

• It is our thermostat

Thanks to more than seven hundred thousand nervous sensors spread out along its entire surface, our skin feels variations in outer temperature and informs the brain of them. The brain in turn transmits to other parts of the body the orders needed to maintain our internal temperature. When it is hot out, we perspire. Small cutaneous blood vessels dilate to evacuate the heat as best they can. A side effect: we turn red. The humidity of the skin helps refresh us, especially when there is a bit of a breeze. Cold provokes the reverse reaction. The cutaneous vessels retract and we grow pale.

The skin and menopause

The skin is sensitive to estrogens and progesterone. Because of the hormone shifts and potential for imbalance at menopause, the skin will have a tendency to become drier, less dense, and wrinkled. It is more sensitive to shock and to the sun. Protect yourself from the sun with a hat and sunscreen. Creams enriched with herbal estrogens and natural progesterone are sold in health food stores, and can help to balance the hormones. Many books are available about this, as well as information on the Internet.

Andropause in men does not have a big effect on the skin, as changes in testosterone level do not affect the skin like estrogen and progesterone fluctuations do. Men will often have an increase in the size of their belly due to testosterone levels dropping off.

• It is an ultra-sensitive envelope

The skin is not only sensitive to touch (even the lightest), but also to the electromagnetic fields around us. Numerous experiments have helped prove that the skin perceives combinations of infrareds, short wave, radio waves, and ultrasounds. Without seeing or touching a person, we can feel his or her presence. For example, one Saturday I was walking in the central square in my city. There were a lot of people. Suddenly I felt a hot wave touch my shoulder, like a close presence. I turned around many times but couldn't see anyone I knew. It turned out to be a friend who was watching me from the fourth floor of a building.

• It is a fat reservoir

When we are deprived of fat in the diet, our body draws on its reserves. Fat is like a cushion to us. What could make sitting on a rock more comfortable than a nicely padded backside? That's just a little joke to draw your attention to the issue of "too much" or "not enough." Fat in excess is unhealthy, but so is too little of it. Fat is the body's way of storing excess energy, so that it can be retrieved later. This process is very efficient. It is regulated in the liver by various hormones but is largely controlled by insulin, the hormone which regulates blood glucose levels. Fat also has a hormonal function, related to the production of estrogens. This explains why women have more sub-cutaneous fat than men—they require more estrogen for their body functions. Overly skinny or anorexic women may have irregular or absent periods and problems becoming pregnant.

• *It is antirachitic (prevents rickets)*

Sun rays (ultraviolet) act upon the cholesterol in the skin, helping it synthesize vitamin D, which in turn (and in tandem with the liver and the kidneys) helps us absorb calcium through digestion. But one should avoid excessive sunbathing between 11 a.m. and 5 p.m. for this can lead to skin cancer.

• *Other people's skin attracts or repels us*

When you touch a person's skin, you pick up a flood of information in only a few seconds. Skin can be smooth, grainy, hairy, thin, thick, hot, fresh, moist, sweaty, etc. It reflects the person's personality, state of health, and emotional state. Skin always has an effect on us. It is a meeting of the flesh with another person, and there will always be a reaction: emotion, attraction, or repulsion. The skin's role is linked to the senses, to relationships, and of course to our sensuality. The contact of one person's skin with another's is always a unique occurrence. It is live sensation. The brain has nothing to do with it.

When the Skin Isn't Working as well as It Should

The skin is our only visible organ. It is reactive and has its ills, large and small. Teenage acne is a common case in point. It is the expression of excessive hormones. Eczema, pimples, dry patches, fungi, dermatitis, impetigo, psoriasis, and herpes are dermatologists' fare. These undesirable symptoms are often reactions to exterior aggressions. Melanoma—cancerous skin tumors due to the sun, or perhaps also to pollution or genetic factors—are more serious.

~Skin People~

Skin people can seem paradoxical: they would like to hide their poor health, stress, or unhappiness, but their skin displays it for all to see. Their characteristics (or, to repeat my earlier explanation of this analysis, the characteristics of the skin as personified in an imaginary archetypal person) include fear of being exposed, withdrawal, timidity, and a feeling of shame. Actually, skin people would like to hide, but their skin problems attract other people's eye. Certain parts of the body are easy to conceal, but others are always exposed. Their skin reflects everything they feel, causing redness, blotches, little cracks, pimples, a cardboard-like or oozing texture, perhaps an unpleasant smell, molten or acid.

Philippe works at a research center for electronic components. The Chamber of Commerce in his city asks him to give a presentation for a large group of industrialists. It's his first conference, and he is both honored and terrified. A week before the event, he has a sudden attack of psoriasis on his neck, hands, and face. He has never had anything like it before. In the family, his grandfather had suffered from psoriasis. Philippe calls to cancel his presentation, but the organizers convince him to lecture. Two weeks after the conference, all trace of psoriasis has disappeared. Philippe's body, under orders from his brain, triggered a skin problem to give him a reason to cancel his appearance at the conference and to let his fear take over.

Following are more traits of skin people.

• *"Feeling good in one's own skin"*

When we're self-confident, "well at ease in our skin" (the French expression is *"bien dans sa peu"*), our skin as well as our general attitude show it. Both are supple and radiant. When we are in good physical and psychological health, our skin is clear and luminous with few or no rough patches or red blotches. The outer showcase of our body and mind reflects

204 ᷳᴖ What Your Organs Think

perfect balance. This is not always the case and it is difficult to hide it. Little pimples caused by liver imbalance, simple blushing due to emotion or sensitivity to the cold—these and other reactions are all but impossible to conceal. We turn red, white, we get goose-bumps—our skin reveals our state of mind through spontaneous emotional reactions.

When we don't feel psychologically "at ease in our skin," our skin itself gives away the signs: psoriasis, pimples, red blotches, dry patches. And conversely, when our skin suffers too much from external physical assaults, we end up feeling ill at ease in our skin.

• Direct emotional connection

Except in the case of spontaneous emotional reactions, the skin acts in correlation with other organs such as the liver, the pancreas, and the lungs. It is an emotional complement in problems such as refusing to be among other people and withdrawing; harboring a fear of contact, whether physical or social; carrying an inferiority complex and engaging in self-deprecation; feeling shame; being shy, reserved, or overly discreet; being hyper-reactive; and needing to be protected.

How to Take Care of the Skin

From a physical and nutritional point of view

The skin is the showcase of our organs. The key to good skin that looks fresh and elastic and is pleasant to the touch is to have well-functioning organs, especially the liver, kidneys, and pancreas. But above all, don't smoke. In our line of work, we can recognize a smoker's skin at a glance: it turns grayish. Tobacco impedes oxygenation of the tissues and makes the skin lose its subtle pinkish hue.

When the kidneys are not working as well as they should, the skin stays creased when you pinch it—in other words, it doesn't recover its shape immediately. It loses some of its elasticity and glow, and gives off a slightly acid smell. When the liver and pancreas are not working as well as they should, the skin oozes. Even after washing it quickly becomes greasy and dull again and has a strong smell, especially under the arms.

Go back to the chapters on each of these organs to see what you can do to improve their functioning.

From a psychological point of view

Skin people tend to feel out of place. They have to learn how to hold themselves up straight, shoulders back and chest forward. It's important for them to look other people in the eye and to avoid looking down; I recommend this to learn how to hold your own. You should try it out initially with people who don't intimidate you. When sitting facing someone, make sure you feel contact with the earth beneath your feet. This solidity is reassuring. If you have serious skin problems, you should see a psychotherapist.

PART THREE

Taking Care of Our Messenger

18

Our Most Precious Possession

As we said in the introduction to this book, we have a duty to monitor our body and health. We were given a natural capital at birth—we should use it but also learn to respect it. When we take good care of ourselves (lifestyle, nutrition, weight), our organs, their "cogwheels" and metabolism, function properly. We obviously feel the benefits. Feeling at ease in our body allows us to feel at ease in our mind. Our physical and psychological beings are in harmony. When we allow little room for illness, depression, or other difficulties to put us off balance, our body and mind are free to enjoy an optimal level of vital energy.

The Quest for Balance

In a world permeated with stress and an environment saturated with chemicals, we urgently need to take special care of our health capital. We need to supply it with the best possible ingredients to achieve physical balance and emotional stability. Our brain records all the emotions and tensions we encounter and redistributes them in our body according to their intensity, setting off superficial or deeper reactions that range from dysfunction to actual illness. Our organs have an ongoing dialogue with our brain. Most of the time the brain receives the emotion and then sends it on to the organs; sometimes—in the case of extreme fear or shock—the nervous system (sympathetic) reacts before the brain, and you can have an instant reaction of an organ (stomach spasm, gallbladder contraction, etc.). Shock accumulates, and when we've undergone one shock too many, however insignificant the most recent one may seem, we can fall ill. Why? Because we have reached our compensation limit, our tolerance threshold. We didn't notice or heed the warning signals, and our body simply could not take any more without damage.

To resist external aggressions and keep them from affecting our body too forcefully, we need to build up a strong "adaptation/compensation" capacity. We go through life like a tightrope walker—we're always trying to keep our balance, so we go forward, leaning slightly to the right, slightly to the left. But if we take a false step and fall, we have to wait for help. Manual therapists who are trained in Visceral Manipulation are here to help us.

Your Health Itinerary

Become aware of the changes in attitude and health that your feelings and emotions create in you. Learn to pinpoint your weaknesses, both physical and psychological.

Your Log Book

If necessary, keep a log. It can be very instructive. For example:

- Today, Friday, stomachache. Yesterday my daughter announced that she was going away by car for the weekend with friends.
- Wednesday, I fell down the stairs. I got very scared. I've had a headache ever since.
- Monday, I feel light as a feather. Great weekend, walk in the forest, picnic, no alcohol or heavy food. Good mood in the family.
- November 1st, All Souls' Day, a pain under my right ribs. Don't feel too great. Thinking about my father, my best friend, all those people who are gone. It's too, too painful!

Like a ship captain, make note of what occurs on board (your body is your boat, it's the vehicle you travel through life with)—jot down when the machines are working efficiently and when there's a technical problem. Whenever you feel the need, you can look through your notes and find explanations or references. The act of writing, of sitting face to face with a sheet of paper (a mirror of our inner self), and concentrating on what we are feeling brings comfort in itself. It's a way of expressing things, reflecting upon them, and understanding them. Excellent psychological work! Some people write down their dreams; don't hesitate to jot down your emotional states and physical sensations. You'll learn how to establish relationships between them and find the meaning behind them. Then you'll start working on avoiding them.

Other ways to connect your body and emotions:

- Understand your inner workings. What type of emotion affects your organs? Which one or ones more specifically? What kind of behavioral or psychological reactions go along with functional imbalance in an organ?
- Determine what your own particular emotion–organ correspondences are, using the models provided in this book.
- Find out which of your organs is your weak link, your greatest emotional catalyst.
- Listen to the alarm signals that your body gives you and to recurrent symptoms.
- Practice working on your emotions and taking care of your organs.

Educating Our Children and Young Athletes

Just as we teach our children respect, politeness, various rules of civility, and other ways to get by in school and in society, we have to teach them the right attitudes to promote their well-being and health. Begin with a few simple but essential principles: eat healthily, sleep well, breathe deeply, move harmoniously. It is useful to have children understand that these few basic habits are just as important for their future as all the learning they're going to absorb at school. Parents who know how to explain and give good advice don't need to forbid. It's a question of plain common sense. Sitting in front of the TV with a bag of potato chips and a pack of candy bars every day is not good for their health. But to go out on a "ketchup and French fries " binge once a week with a bunch of friends is a treat and it's great, because sharing the fun helps prevent compulsive or addictive attitudes. Rules of good balance learned and applied from the youngest age will inevitably bear fruit over the long term. If our children are raised learning to take care of their health capital, then later on, as adults, they'll know how to make correct choices concerning their job, lifestyle, environment, and health. "Good living" is an acquired ability!

Young athletes need to adopt a particularly healthy lifestyle as a basis for their daily regimen. It's not enough to be talented, strong, and well-trained. Nutritional balance and good sleeping habits are also important fuel for good performance. To be attentive and kind to our body is to grant our physical and mental energy its full power—the power of champions.

Respecting the Balance Within Our Body

We have no control over our genetics or our age. We are the victims of the pollution in our environment, the anxiety of our times, stress in our profession.... But we can act to limit the harmful effects on our health capital. We are ultimately our own doctor. We can promote our well-being through:

- psychological balance (dealing with our emotions, exercising)
- physical balance (activity, exercise)
- respecting our natural rhythms (sleep, breathing)
- nutritional balance (giving our motor better-quality fuel: food and drink)
- the pleasures of life (travels, friends, outings, art, shows...).

Psychological Balance

Dealing with our emotions. When an emotion arises, there are two ways of dealing with it. One is to objectify our emotional reaction by holding someone or something responsible for our state. This method reinforces and intensifies negative feelings. The other solution is to dive deep into the emotion itself, to discover it, feel every aspect of it, 'become' this emotion and calmly observe our own nature. The text *Time, Space and Knowledge* by Tarthang Tulku, a Tibetan monk, shows us the way of the Buddhist or Zen attitude, from which our serenity and health can profit greatly.

Emotion hits us. It enters our body and mind. It is very present. We can't avoid it—this is only normal! We are all human. We have feelings and reactions. But they are not always easy to bear, because along with the emotion, we receive a number of parasitic phenomena (faster heartbeat, visceral reactions, chaotic thought processes, uncontrolled decisions...) which disturb our inner balance. So instead of kindling the fire within us, we might learn to appease it. It is bad for our well-being to dwell over things, to be angry at perpetrators or agitators, at events and at life in general. All these attitudes feed and increase anxiety. Knowing how to control our emotions, how to observe them instead of being carried away by them, gives us a chance to rapidly regain our peace and positive dynamics of body and mind.

You should know that you can spare yourselves the pain attached to emotion—or at least tame it, and thereby protect your body. An emotion is like a cat. A domesticated cat will purr and let you pet it. This cat is a soothing friend. A wild cat will be aggressive and scratch you. That cat is an enemy who can give you "cat's claw" disease—a real nuisance. Overwhelming emotions need to be expressed, but it's not easy. Society demands that we keep silent about certain emotions. So we have to find personal solutions to help diminish our emotional tensions, such as practicing relaxation, visualization, yoga ... or if necessary, seeing a therapist (see page 224).

Take your time to think things over. Never act under the impulse of an emotion. Avoid letting yourself get carried away and making hasty decisions. It is important to give things time so as to avoid regret for our actions. Indeed, everything is relative, and what may seem insurmountable today may be much less so tomorrow. "It's best to sleep on it," as the saying goes. The time we take to reflect allows the emotion to die down, and gives us a chance to analyze the situation more clearly, to sort out all the different elements and eliminate the negative ones, so that we can build on the basis of the more positive ones.

Take on a Zen attitude. You probably put a lot of care into decorating and keeping up your intimate surroundings (your house or apartment). You should put just as much care into seeking your own inner harmony. Harmony is to be found in ourselves as much as in our home. Let positive energy circulate in your mind as well as in your living quarters. Gentleness, clarity, transparency, but also movement, colors, vibrations. Cultivate your inner beauty as well as your *"savoir vivre"*—the art of good living. Practice yoga, relaxation, meditation, or tai-chi. Learn to laugh at yourself. Sometimes it's best to "make light of it."

Physical Balance

Respect your body. Respecting your body means being attentive to how it is functioning and answering its needs. This will guarantee you healthy senior years: you'll be as dynamic at seventy as you were at twenty. Take control of your health and well-being. Listen to your own common sense and be mindful of foods or habits which do not agree with you. Observe your reactions and make a note of whatever does not agree with you, so you can avoid it in the future.

Get moving! Exercising helps you get rid of your stress, empty out your mind, recharge your batteries, lose weight, and improve your cardiac function. It is also very good for your mental health. The endorphins that your body produces during exercise promote a state of well-being. Movement brings oxygen to your muscles and brain, helping you feel at home in your body and experience a true sense of being alive. The more mastery you gain over your movements, the more you'll enjoy exercising—alone, with friends, or with the family. The simple act of walking is enough to establish a healthy balance.

If you're not inclined to doing sports, walk briskly at least half an hour a day, without overdoing it or exhausting yourself, ideally in a pleasant area out in the fresh air, so that you'll be tempted to do it again. Once you have felt the benefits of being physically active, you'll want to try swimming, aerobic classes, or why not a bit of cross-country running! You'll end up saying: enough of being a couch potato! Certain sports such as Pilates and dancing teach you to coordinate your movements and reinforce your sense of balance. Cross-country running on a supple terrain and bicycling—except in rare cases of medical contraindication—are among the secrets of longevity. We have tested the tension in many people's bodies before and after exercising. The differences are amazing. The muscles relax, the organs are more supple and are less sensitive when we palpate them The facial features are also more relaxed. Getting involved in pleasurable exercise is really worth the effort! Human beings are made to move.

The Balance of Rhythms

Our organs function according to certain rhythms, which are not the same for everyone. Learning to know and respect them is giving ourselves the benefit of extra "health assets." A balanced way of life requires that we pay attention to our biorhythmic nature. Whether it be eating, sleeping, or other rhythms, you'll hear remarks such as "I work like a clock" or, at the other extreme, "My body is totally out of sync." A well-oiled machine is one that receives proper care from its happy owner. It's just a question of listening to our body and to ourselves!

We each have our own rhythm. According to Oriental medicine, we are all subject to our own biorhythms, and we are also influenced by external rhythms. Energy circulates through our organs following a circadian (approximately 24 hours) rhythm: it begins in the lungs, between 3 and 5 a.m., goes through the colon between 5 and 7 a.m., then the stomach and ends up in the liver from 1 to 3 a.m., returning to the lungs. Our organism is subject to this circadian rhythm, but also to monthly cycles (the ovarian cycle, for example) and annual ones.

Our tolerance threshold. It is best to lead a well-ordered (which does not mean boring) life, respecting our natural rhythms and permitting ourselves a bit of leeway once in a while, just for the fun of it! Accumulating stress and excesses is what harms your body. If you feel you've gone beyond your limits, that you can no longer take those sleepless nights, those destabilizing changes in schedule, that intense stress that is disturbing your respiratory or digestive system, it is time to slow down. See a specialist (relaxation therapist, psychotherapist, homeopath, etc.; see page 224). He or she will help you phase back into your biological rhythms and regain your balance.

Sleep

Sleep is part of our health capital. It has a repairing function. If it is deficient in quantity or quality and doesn't fulfill our body's requirements, functional disharmony will ensue. Our vital energy is no longer properly maintained. This can affect our nervous, cardiovascular and/or digestive systems. What counts above all is the quality of our sleep. We don't all have the same needs in terms of quantity: some people feel great after only five or six hours' sleep; other people need eight or even nine hours. Some are night birds and don't go to bed before midnight, but don't ask them to get up at dawn; others are morning birds and their minds are ticking away as early as 6 a.m., but don't ask them to stay up too late at night. We all have our own personal clock. The main thing is to respect it as far as duration (length of sleep) is concerned, as well as your ideal bedtime and rising time. In any case, the first hours of sleep are the most important ones. They constitute a deep sleep phase which brings the most repair physically and psychologically. Sometimes there can be difficulties:

- *Couples who don't share the same sleep cycles:* They will necessarily conflict. It's not always easy to adapt.
- *People who are obsessed with sleep.* They are convinced they will awaken tired and therefore begin going to bed earlier and earlier, counting the hours spent in bed, some of which are unfortunately passed rehashing yesterday's problems, instead of benefiting from restful sleep.
- *Daytime nap aficionados:* Too long a nap will alter the quality of nighttime sleep, whereas a brief half-hour rest is beneficial.

The Organs and Sleep

Dysfunction in an organ will often affect our sleep.

The digestive system. We all know that after too heavy a meal or too much alcohol, it's not easy to sleep well. We're restless, fretful, we feel hot and thirsty and have bad dreams....

The liver and the pancreas. People who go to bed around 10 p.m., for example, might wake up suddenly around 1 or 2 a.m., perspiring so heavily that they have to remove the covers to reduce their body temperature. It will be impossible for them to fall back asleep on their right side. These nightly disturbances are often due to over-rich meals: too sweet or too fatty, or too much alcohol. The temperature in certain veins in the liver goes up to 104°F during digestion.

The stomach. It sounds its alarm at about 4 or 5 a.m. People will feel heartburn or pain in the upper and middle part of their stomach, and around the ribs on the left side. They can't sleep on their stomach and will fall back asleep more comfortably on their right side.

The bronchial passages. They wake sleepers up around the same hours as the stomach. Smokers will cough and need to spit out phlegm; asthmatic people will have trouble breathing.

The kidneys. When congested, they'll disturb sleep between 4 and 7 a.m. Often the simple act of emptying the bladder alleviates tension in the kidneys. Kidney problems often bring on a backache upon awakening which eases in the course of the morning.

Keeping a Nutritional Balance

Nutritional balance is based on rather simple rules. The key word is "adapting"—adapting our nutrition to our body's needs. But the problem is learning to understand and know our needs. "Let your food be your medicine" said Hippocrates, the Father of Medicine. Food is a natural medicine: it helps the body stay in good shape, and to fight off stress and illness. Its intake has to be well managed, but eating should remain a pleasure, based on common sense.

Nutritional habits can be disconcerting. Two squares of chocolate are excellent to keep in good cheer, but to gobble down a whole bar guarantees an upset stomach, at least for some people. We must learn to enjoy in moderation. Excesses often come from behavioral problems. The cumulative effect can be a catastrophe for the body: "Two croissants a day isn't that much, but by the end of the year, that's 730! No small matter for the digestive system!" says a renowned French chef.

Major food companies, whose aim is to make profit by attracting new customers and making sure that "older" ones keep buying, invent addictive products. Sweet sodas are slightly salted to make you thirsty again. You drink one and you crave another one! Addiction to industrial beverages and foods (potato chips, chocolate bars, pastry, and so on) is a frequent problem in young people, especially in the United States, where the number of obese people is frightening—almost thirty percent of the population. Even in France, the figures are rising rapidly.

Digestion: not always logical. As we all know, with digestion we tend to have one good day followed by a not so good day. One morning you'll wake up feeling sick to your stomach although you had nothing outrageous to eat the night before. Food is not the only factor which acts upon proper digestive function. Other very subtle parameters play a role:

- the season
- the time
- the hormone cycle
- the state of stress you're in
- physical effort
- the company you share while eating
- sleep

Certain foods aid digestion and others disturb it and can even be toxic. They are not the same for everybody. Tolerance or rejection depends on each person's digestive sensitivity. The level of acidity in the stomach varies according to the time of day. Before their period, many women have trouble digesting heavy or fatty foods. It is said that white peaches are excellent for the liver, but they don't agree with some people—these are just a couple of examples to show that digestion has its secrets.

How to recognize which foods agree with you

- You digest them easily and quickly.
- You enjoy eating them. You enjoy their taste, smell, consistency, and feel.
- You feel well and light after eating something.

It's a matter of common sense!

Fruits and Vegetables

There are very few vegetables that are not recommended to everyone.

- People who are prone to fermentation in the intestines should eat their vegetables cooked. They are much easier to digest.
- Allergies to certain fruits or vegetables do exist. In such cases, the particular foods must be avoided. But before incriminating the food itself, check its origin and how it was treated. Certain commonly used chemicals can cause allergies. The nitrate that is present in water is a typical example. Nitrates irritate the digestive tube, causing hypersensitivity in the intestinal mucous membranes, which in turn can induce allergies. When a mucous membrane is irritated or congested, it will become the prey of all allergy factors: pollution, stress, poor eating habits, etc.

Watch out for these foods:

- *Tomatoes:* If you are not sure of their origin, remove the skin.
- *Carrots:* Buy them whole and grate them yourself.

- *Oranges:* If their skin is very shiny, they've been chemically treated. Choose oranges that are not too sour and make fresh juice for breakfast. Avoid eating them in the afternoon and evening.
- *Grapes:* Careful, they are often heavily sprayed. If you can't buy organic, wash them thoroughly, or even soak them in a bowl of water for a while. Dark muscat grapes are excellent for the intestines and kidneys.
- *Prunes:* Watch out for sulfites. Read the label carefully. Prunes contain sorbitol, which is a natural digestive aid.
- *Apples:* Choose them carefully, checking where they are from and how they've been treated. Select apples from small farms where the fruit is treated as little as possible and only with natural products. You'll find them in markets or health food stores. When they are slightly sour, they're an aid to digestion. When they are too mealy, they're more difficult to digest.

The chemical industry is a very powerful lobby, compared to those of us preoccupied with "eating healthily." One of my patients, an apple grower, explained to me how the fruit in his groves ripens: "I use pesticides and insecticides, just like everybody else. When I spray the apples on the tree, I now wear gloves and a mask: two of my workers developed skin diseases. I pick them green and store them in cold rooms, at 40°F. I gas them with ethylene and then with carbon dioxide." He adds candidly, "It's not dangerous and doesn't change the appearance of the fruit. The apples are smooth and firm."

Scary, isn't it? Remember that a spotless fruit is a dangerous fruit.

Beneficial Foods

- *Onion:* In small quantities, it stimulates the liver. In large quantities, it causes gas.
- *Garlic:* An excellent antioxidant. Good for the intestines, it has an anti-parasite effect. If you have animals at home, make sure you eat garlic once in a while.

- *Leek:* Contains a lot of magnesium. It's good for the liver and the pancreas because it slows down the assimilation of simple carbohydrates. It's a digestive aid.
- *Mâche (Lamb's Lettuce):* Recommended for the liver and the gallbladder. It contains omega-3s.
- *Spinach, rhubarb:* Good for the intestines. Watch out, your stomach may react to their acidity (especially with rhubarb).
- *Dandelion:* Good for the liver, pancreas, and gallbladder.
- *Celery:* Good for the liver.
- *Black radish:* Good for the gallbladder and the liver. I highly recommend it.
- *Ginseng:* Good for the liver and pancreas. But too much will irritate the stomach. It is also known as an aphrodisiac.
- *Potatoes:* They contain vitamin C. There are countless varieties. La Ratte potatoes, for instance, are a delicacy!
- *Artichoke:* Good for the liver and the gallbladder. It can cause fermentation in the intestines. In that case, change the water twice while cooking them and rinse them once they are cooked.
- *Fennel:* Good for the liver and gallbladder. Add little bits raw in salad. It's excellent for digestion.
- *Endives:* Good for the kidneys and stomach.
- *Peppers:* Raw, they stimulate the digestive function. Cooked they can be hard to digest, depending on how they are prepared.
- *Grapefruit:* Good for the liver and the gallbladder. Avoid canned juice.
- *Lemon:* A few drops in lukewarm water are excellent for the kidneys, and in the morning for the gallbladder and the liver. But a whole glass will irritate the stomach.
- *Pineapple:* Fresh, of course. At the end of a meal, it helps digestion. Good for the pancreas, the liver, and the lungs.

- *Blackberries:* In small quantities, they stimulate the liver.
- *Redcurrant:* Good for the pancreas in small quantities. Their sourness can irritate the stomach.
- *Kiwi:* It contains vitamin C, but its reputation is slightly overrated. Good for the intestines.
- *White peaches:* Good for the liver and intestines.
- *Blueberries:* Good for the stomach. They enhance the eyesight. Royal Air Force pilots used to eat blueberry jam to be able to see better at night.
- *Tangerines:* Good for the intestines. Don't buy them too sour, or they could irritate the stomach.

Fats

Oils. When we buy oil, we think we're getting pure grain or fruit extract. Unfortunately, this is not the case with certain oils. The grains are cleansed, ground, and heated. Refined oils often contain additives: solvents, acids, phosphates, soda, bleaching agents, food coloring.... This is because the more you heat the grains or fruits, the more oil can be extracted. But the balance of its ingredients will be consequently offset. By choosing "extra virgin cold-pressed" oils, you can be sure of their quality. "Cold-pressed" does not really mean "cold": the oil is pressed at around 95 to 105°F. Olive or peanut oil are best for frying.

Omega-3 and omega-6. Omega-3s (alpha-linoleic acid) and omega-6s (linolenic acid) are fats that the body metabolizes easily but does not produce itself. Therefore you should make sure you are getting enough of them. They are considered to have anti-thrombosis, anti-atheromatous, and anti-inflammatory virtues. Omega-3s are found particularly in canola, walnut, and hazelnut oil; omega-6s in olive and sunflower seed oil (also very rich in vitamin E). Walnut and hazelnut oil also contain omega-6, vitamin E, and lecithin (found in soy and egg yoke as well). Lecithin is good for the heart, brain, nervous system, liver, and pancreas.

Butter. Traditionally, it takes twenty-two quarts of milk to make 2.2 pounds of butter. In principle, no additives, food colorings, or preservatives are used. It is the grass the cow grazes that gives the butter a lighter or darker color. The more chlorophyll and beta-carotene the grass contains, the darker the butter. Butter contains a lot of vitamin A. Have a little at breakfast on your bread—that will cover your daily requirements.

Water, Only Water!

No water, no life! Our body is made up of approximately seventy percent water (the percentage is higher when we are born and typically decreases as we age). The water's role is to dilute and to filter. It is sensitive to variations in atmospheric pressure and humidity. According to the altitude, the season, food (and beverage), the water in our body is subject to variable pressure.

The influence of the lunar cycle. Under the influence of lunar attraction, the tide moves billions of cubic feet of water. It would be surprising if the water in our body were not submitted to the same phenomenon. This could explain what sometimes seem like mysterious variations in how we feel. Woodcutters and carpenters used to cut wood according to the moon cycle. "Cut with a waxing moon, and the boards don't warp and are less prone to parasites," they would say, and it seems they were right.

Water circulates in our organs. Our organs secrete about two gallons of water per day:

- saliva: 1 to 1.5 quarts a day
- stomach: 2 to 3 quarts a day
- pancreas: 1.5 quarts a day
- liver: 1 quart a day
- intestines: 2 to 3 quarts a day
- bronchial tubes: 1 quart a day

The cerebrospinal fluid also needs water. It surrounds the brain and the spinal cord, nourishing and protecting them.

These figures prove that we must drink to ensure proper functioning of our organs. Drink regularly, often, but a little at a time. If you swallow too much water at once, the water absorbed by the stomach comes right back out as sweat. In winter, it goes directly into the bladder, too quickly to leave the kidneys enough time to eliminate toxins. Conversely, if the body lacks water, it will become intoxicated. The urine becomes too concentrated and can even produce kidney stones. Watch out for water that contains too much sodium, especially sparkling water. Some brands contain twenty times more salt than others. Check the label. Salt retains water in the body, causing congestion and swelling, and raises the blood pressure.

Conclusion: Let's drink, but intelligently. Let's eat, but moderately.

How Complementary and Alternative Medicine Can Help Us

As long as we can, we must do without sleeping pills, tranquilizers, or antidepressant medicine. They may help us through times of low functioning, but they don't solve the problem and can even be harmful to our health. Let's not fool ourselves: a person who is a threat to him- or herself or to other people will not be helped with a bit of relaxation or homeopathy—something more extreme and immediate is necessary. In such cases, allopathy is more than recommended. But it's a long way before we reach such a state, and there are various therapy methods which are a complement to allopathic medicine and can be of great help: manual therapies such as Visceral Manipulation and Nerve Manipulation, acupuncture, sophrology (see below), Bach flowers, homeopathy, psychotherapy, yoga, and more.

Listen to your body, listen to your intuition.

Choose Your Therapist Carefully

- First of all, you should have the feeling that he or she understands you. A relationship between two people is based on unconscious and subtle immediate perceptions, and not only on verbal communication. If you don't "get a good feeling" from the therapist, it will surely work both ways.
- The number of sessions should be based on simple logic and on a moral agreement. You are working together

to facilitate your healing. The therapist is not doing it to you; you must participate. There must be honest communication between you and the therapist to ensure optimal treatment. The therapist must also be able to communicate if they feel they have helped you all they can and refer you to another practitioner. In the case of physical pain, if you don't feel any benefit after three or four sessions, something is wrong. Either the type of therapy is not beneficial for your condition, the therapist is not skilled enough to assist you, or you many be doing things that are decreasing the effectiveness of the treatment. What you do physically, nutritionally, and mentally between therapy sessions plays a major role in the success of your treatments. Remember you have your body for many more hours a day than you are receiving therapy. It may take more than the three or four sessions for the situation to fully resolve, but you should see progress by then. When it comes to the psyche, the number of sessions is harder to establish. But you should feel there is a plan, a therapeutic project.

- If the therapy you chose isn't showing the desired results, the therapist should take the initiative and redirect you toward a more suitable type of therapy. A good therapist should be able to feel very quickly if the techniques he or she is using are going to bear fruit or not.

- Remember that nobody "belongs" to any therapist. You are free.

- For the therapist, the issue must be to improve the patient's health, and not to get a grip on the person. If there is any doubt or if the patient loses trust in the therapist, he or she should not hesitate to see someone else.

- A therapist should keep his or her place, and not judge you or your family and friends. Avoid those who make you feel guilty, who mix religion and therapy, or who ask you to join a group. Abuse does occur, you can easily detect it from the onset if you don't let yourself get caught up in anything.

Efficient alternative solutions. Specialists will tell you all about them. Among the many different kinds of alternative medicine, we've chosen to explain four in some detail below. This does not mean that other methods are not equally efficient.

Visceral Manipulation Therapy

This field addresses all aspects of our body, from head to toe. Our limited space here will only allow us to touch upon a few of the most frequent types of Visceral Manipulation, which belong to the manual therapist's therapeutic kit. They make it possible to increase an organ's mobility and improve its functioning. There are specific techniques for every organ. By favoring visceral mobility, the manual therapist can break the vicious "emotion-organ-behavior" circle that maintains emotional, psychological, and physical imbalance. The manual therapist can act to the benefit of your organs.

The kidneys. During pregnancy, the baby often has a tendency to compress the kidneys or the ureters (tubes that lead from the kidneys to the bladder), which sometimes causes kidney infections (pyelonephritis), hypertension, lumbago, or sciatica. A manual therapist can teach a pregnant woman postures that help prevent such problems and allow the baby to be less compressed. If you are pregnant, I particularly recommend this exercise:

In an "Arab prayer position" (on your knees, upper body and head bent forward, your arms stretched out in front of you, and the palms of your hands on the floor), let go of your tummy when breathing in and push it inwards when breathing out. Repeat the movement several times, taking care not to arch your spine.

This posture gives the baby space while relieving the kidneys, sciatic nerve, and vena cava from the compression. The vena cava is a large vein in the stomach area that branches out into several other veins which go into the legs. Compression of the vena cava can cause varicose veins, especially on the left side.

The liver and gallbladder. When the gallbladder is prone to producing gallstones, a manual therapist can help empty it using specific Visceral Manipulations. He or she can also work on a congested liver or a hardened and less mobile liver, following hepatitis. Visceral Manipulation is very helpful to the liver, and the person usually feels the benefit immediately.

The stomach. Hiatal hernia and reflux are related to the liver. Therefore, a manual therapist will work on the liver to achieve an effect on the junction between the esophagus and the stomach. Through Visceral Manipulation, a manual therapist can relieve the pain caused by an ulcer, as a complement to the medicine which keeps the patient comfortable. But it's mainly after the ulcer has been cured or after an operation that the manual therapist can prevent scar adhesions from forming, thanks to very specific movements. A stomach that is too low down (yes, this does happen!) can't empty out properly. Its acidity level rises, and the bile and pancreatic juices sometimes flow back into the stomach, instead of on into the intestine and duodenum. A manual therapist can help the stomach find a better position, and make it more mobile and functional.

The intestine. See a manual therapist for Visceral Manipulation after any surgery in the abdomen: he or she can locate and free scar adhesions. They are almost always present. Depending on where they are located, they can cause intestinal problems, including a risk of intestinal blockage or vein and lymph circulation problems. At the lower end of the intestine, adhesions can affect the bladder and uterus.

The thorax and its contents. In the event of serious trauma (a fall on the back, a car or bicycle accident, a fall off a horse, etc.), we all tend to think of the spine and to forget the ribs and everything that is inside the thorax. A manual therapist will pay special attention to these supposedly secondary areas in your body. It is also useful to see a manual therapist after a heart or lung operation. He or she will check the state of your ribs, diaphragm, pleura, and heart attachments.

The genital organs. Retroversion (tilting) of the uterus can cause circulation problems in the pelvis and legs, as well as lower back pain. A manual therapist will not try to change the position of a uterus; it will unfailingly move back into retroversion again. Visceral Manipulation's purpose will be to restore mobility and proper functioning to the uterus and cervix. Regular walking also helps the uterus maintain its mobility. The small canals in the fallopian tubes become obstructed very easily following unnoticed micro-infections. This sometimes leads to infertility. Thanks to very gentle manipulations, a manual therapist can stretch the fallopian tubes to make them more passable. We must remain reserved and prudent as to the results, but certain patients are convinced that they were able to have a child thanks to Visceral Manipulation.

Freeing emotions through the organs. Certain techniques make it possible to get rid of emotional baggage stored in the organs. By laying one hand on the organ and the other on the patient's head, the manual therapist can release tensions by exerting very light pressure. When properly used, these techniques can produce astonishing results, if whatever mechanical tensions were present were taken care of first.

Acupuncture

(SECTION CONTRIBUTED BY DOMINIQUE THÉVENOT, ACUPUNCTURIST AND OSTEOPATH)

Acupuncture is one of the techniques used in traditional Chinese medicine, which is thought to go back as far as several centuries before the current era. It combines remedies (herbal medicine), specific energetic exercises (chi-gong), dietetics, massages, and the freeing of certain joints with its famed needle techniques. The techniques are chosen after a diagnosis has been established according to the traditional Chinese approach. The diagnosis has nothing to do with diagnosis in our Western medicine. It is established with following procedures:

- a very detailed series of questions (similar in precision to a homeopath's)
- examination of the tongue (color, coating, shape)
- examination of the complexion

• taking different pulses. Through digital palpation, the
therapist determines the depth, tension, power, rhythm,
quality, and proper location of the arterial pulse. The
pulse is taken in the wrists, feet, groin, neck, and head.

Once the imbalance has been identified, the therapist will choose the
approach that seems most suitable for the patient. Acupuncture, herbal
medicine, energetic exercise—all result from the same diagnosis and the
same therapeutic laws. If the therapist chooses acupuncture, he or she
will determine which points to work on according to a system established through meticulous observation of the laws of nature and in analogy with them: hot, cold, humid, dry, day, night, heaven, earth, all the
different energies—in short, yin and yang. These laws are called, among
others, "the law of the five elements" or "the six qualities of heaven." For
example, a urinary infection triggered by an annoying event can be treated (in certain patients) through points in the liver meridian, if the pulse
and interrogation confirm this diagnosis. For other patients, whose pulse
reveals an imbalance in the bladder, the therapist will choose totally different points, such as kidney or bladder points.

The points are sort of like floodgates, located on or in (sometimes on
and in) energetic paths called the meridians. The acupuncturist stimulates them with very fine needles—or through heat, with moxa sticks
(little artemisia sticks which are burnt either directly on the skin or at
a slight distance from the skin so as to act upon reflex zones or specific
areas of the skin)—at very specific depths, so as to connect different parts
of the body with the organs and influence their physiology. The meridians and points are not based on specific anatomical areas, but sometimes
they face or are near key points in the vascular or nervous system.

Illness, poor health, fatigue, fainting, and psychosomatic or "somato-
psychological" disturbances are all indications that the body's automatic
regulation system is not functioning in a satisfactory manner. You have to
change from automatic to manual shifting, like a sailor who takes the rud-
der in his hand when the automatic pilot has shut down! An acupuncturist

will treat a person or simply a symptom, but not the illness *per se*. This makes acupuncture especially helpful in so-called functional disturbances, with symptoms such as insomnia, headaches, vertigo, palpitations, nausea, digestive problems, asthma, allergies, period irregularities, various aches and pains, fatigue following serious illnesses, etc.

There are hardly any contraindications to acupuncture—perhaps a couple of "non-indications." For example, it would be very hard to help a person who is on the verge of collapse through acupuncture alone. Just like homeopathy and manual therapy, acupuncture helps the patient's constitution and physiology regain its innate potential for health. This is why it can be said that it is particularly recommended as a preventive therapy.

Sophrology

(SECTION CONTRIBUTED BY MARYVONNE TROUILLON, SOPHROLOGIST)

Sophrology is a science, a way of life, and a philosophy all in one. It aims at restoring a balance between the three main aspects of our personality: mind, body, and behavior.

To achieve this, it works on our states and levels of consciousness using different techniques:

- Becoming aware of and learning how to practice good, deep abdominal breathing.
- "Letting go" and developing positive awareness through words, images, and feelings.
- Freeing oneself from daily stress through appropriate exercises and becoming aware of the present moment: "Here and now."

The purpose of sophrology is to help the person become as autonomous as possible. Sophrology is practiced throughout Europe, but it is not common as a separate modality in the U.S. Many manual therapists incorporate similar techniques in their practice and share this information as "homework" for the client. There are a lot of books and information on the Internet about breathing exercises, positive thinking, imagery, and stress-releasing exercises.

Bach Flower Remedies

(SECTION CONTRIBUTED BY DR. FRANÇOISE COULLET,
MEMBER OF THE REGISTER OF THE BACH FOUNDATION)

Bach flowers are preparations distilled from flowers; their purpose is to restore an emotional balance. Doctor Edward Bach, a British homeopath and biologist, devoted his entire life to looking in nature for a way to treat illness gently, painlessly, and without danger. His numerous clinical observations proved the importance of the patient's emotional state and personality in treating his or her illness. A human being is born with a set of emotional characteristics which make up his or her basic "equipment," as necessary to life as the body's organs. Doctor Bach discovered medical uses for thirty-eight different flowers that he linked to thirty-eight emotional states. He divided them into seven groups which fit the main disturbances he encountered: fear, loneliness, lack of interest in the present, doubt, hypersensitivity, discouragement, excessive preoccupation with other people.

These floral elixirs can bring about harmony by removing emotional blockage. Each floral preparation counterbalances a negative emotion and gently restores the patient's balance. The flowers influence the patient's physical health via his or her psychological state. Bach flowers do not treat a disease but a patient as a whole, independently of his or her clinical symptoms. Recognizing the specific emotional state is the keystone of Bach flower diagnosis. A patient's flower "profile" is determined mainly by talking with the person. A therapy with no undesirable side effects, it can be applied to patients of any age, from birth to old age. This therapeutic approach is recommended in a wide variety of cases, along two main axis: either in a specific situation such as a particular difficulty in life, mourning, illness, etc.; or to help a patient discern positive elements in his or her life and develop self-awareness.

Other Therapies

Psychoanalysis. It helps resolve conflicts by looking at our past, reliving it, analyzing it, and interpreting it. In the course of analysis, subconscious elements emerge and can be expressed through words and actions. The patient frees him- or herself from psychological problems through transference on the analyst. In this way past conflicts can be "worked out" in the present.

Psychotherapy. Based on verbal exchange with the psychotherapist, this therapy—in which words are very important—makes it possible to analyze facts and situations, helping the patient resolve conflicts. Psychotherapy is easier for some patients to accept than psychoanalysis.

Behavioral therapy. Through appropriate exercises, this approach helps the person analyze his or her problem and find better solutions. This type of therapy is based on learning and conditioning.

Chi-gong. Literally meaning "energy work," this Chinese practice is based on movement and helps get the energy flowing in the body. It is an energetic form of relaxation, derived from Chinese philosophy and traditional medicine.

Shiatsu. With this Japanese massage and pressure method, the Shiatsu practitioner uses his or her hands and fingers help release blockage and get the energy circulating in the body. In Europe, it is particularly popular in Italy.

Yoga. This is another practice linked to energy flow. It is based on postures, concentration, and relaxation achieved through breath control.

Eutony and Alexander Technique. These methods are different, but similar, and lead to relaxation and freedom of movement, through postures and stretching. They also include work on internalization. Eutony is not well-known in the U.S., while Alexander Technique is more common.

There are countless "gentle" methods to help improve your well-being. We might also mention:

- Aromatherapy, based on essential oils.
- Micro-physical therapy, which awakens the body's memory.

- T'ai chi ch'uan, combining a martial art, gymnastics, and meditation in very slow movement sequences.
- Stretching, which helps eliminate tensions by achieving greater suppleness.
- Visualizing one's problems: the person works through a situation in his or her mind.
- Meditation, often hard to practice!
- The Mézières method, comprised of stretching exercises which activate the entire body.
- Massage and balneo-therapy (hydrotherapy) are also some of the well-being techniques we can turn to today.
- Trace elements, vitamin, and mineral supplements are excellent "better-being" strategies, but it's best to see your therapist to make the right choices.
- And let's not forget dancing, music, drawing, painting, and all forms of artistic expression.

More about Visceral Manipulation

Are There Specific Therapies for Our Organs?

We have seen throughout this book that a good diet, regular exercise, and expressing our emotions are good things to do to feel better in our life. But are there specific treatments that can directly help our organs? Acupuncture, Homeopathy, Massage, Spa, Hammam, Sauna—these are all popular therapies that are known to contribute to our health. However, the therapy known as "Visceral Manipulation" has been shown to be one of the best in optimizing our organ function.

What Is Visceral Manipulation?

Our organs are in perpetual motion. When you breathe, when you walk, when you run, when you stretch yourself, your organs move in your thorax (chest area) and in your abdomen. During normal activity, your diaphragm moves 24,000 times a day to accomplish breathing. Imagine how much more it moves when you exercise or do other strenuous activities. What this also means is that when everything is functioning correctly, the abdominal organs can move a minimum of two thousand feet a day. For example, during normal activity the kidneys move about one inch during inhalation, and they do that in three dimensions! With a deep breath they can move four inches, and that is just in the up and down motion! In reality, they also rotate and bend sideways. What this translates to in a day is moving a distance just over half a mile. Throughout your entire life, your kidneys will each move a distance of approximately 19,000 miles. That is not quite the distance around the Earth (25,000 miles), but close. That's impressive!

Are All Our Organs Moving?

Yes, they all move but at different speeds, in various directions, and with variable timing. The lungs, liver, spleen, pancreas, and intestines are all moving with the diaphragm. The pelvic organs move with the diaphragm much of the time, but they are more dependent on the activity of our legs; this includes activities of the bladder and the rectum, the urinary and intestinal filling and evacuating, and for women the menstrual cycles, pregnancy, and delivery. But remember when you walk, run, or stretch all your organs move also and therefore require good mobility.

The heart has a small movement all its own. It is a kind of torsion whereby the lower part rotates on itself (imagine a toy top that is able to move in various directions all the while standing on its point). At the same time it beats 100,000 times a day!

The brain has tiny movements as well. For example, it glides a little when you bend forward. In the case of an accident, it makes tiny but violent movements inside the skull, which can cause a concussion or coma, or destroy the neurons.

What Is the Purpose of These Movements?

In order for a person to be healthy, all of the numerous elements (organs, muscles, blood, etc.) must have proper motion. For example, proper mobility of the blood helps the organs to accomplish their different functions such as digestion, circulation, immunity, and hormonal production. Some physiologists say that aging is the act of losing our elasticity, mobility, and flexibility. Rigidity is the beginning of poor health.

Our internal system is very complicated, and the more we learn, the more aware we become of the limits of our knowledge. To move is indispensable. When you walk, run, stretch, or do sports, you do more than you realize. You activate all of your body physiology.

How Does Visceral Manipulation Therapy Work?

What are visceral manipulations? As we discussed, each organ has a specific movement pattern when it is healthy. Due to such things as injuries, poor posture, and emotional traumas, organs can lose some or all of this important motion. Visceral Manipulation enable the organs to regain or improve their mobility. This is done using gentle and precise pressure and movements. The therapist first analyzes the body to find visceral fixations. This means areas where the organ doesn't move correctly. The fingers of the therapist "speak" to the tissues, which contain all of your story.

The therapist is also looking to determine why the organs are not moving optimally. For example, the therapist finds a little scar due to infection, trauma, or surgery. The therapist will apply a little movement to very precisely stretch the adhesion. The reason is it important to treat the adhesion is that it irritates some of the small nerves, which produces a spasm in some of the organs like the stomach, the intestines, or the gallbladder. In other organs it will provoke a spasm of some of the adjacent arteries, thereby diminishing the capacity of the organs to play their role correctly.

What Are the Causes of Loss of Mobility?

There are so many reasons for an organ to lose its mobility: sedentary lifestyle, physical traumas, surgery (even colonoscopy), infections, bad diet, pollution, pregnancy, delivery, and so on. For instance, low back pain during pregnancy is seldom due to lumbar spine or disc problems. In fact, most of the time it's due to compression of the kidneys by the baby. The best way to improve this is to ask the expectant mother to do some exercises when on all fours. This will decrease the pressure on the abdominal organs which is caused by the growing baby.

When you fall down on the coccyx or experience an impact during a car accident, high dense organs like the liver, the kidneys, or the spleen receive and store part of the energy produced by the trauma. Sometimes it is difficult for the patient to see the correlation between the trauma and the pain they are having because the symptoms will appear much later.

Can an Organ Be Displaced?

Yes, but this is not very common. The radiologist knows very well that the kidneys can be found several centimeters lower than usual; this is called kidney ptosis. This may cause some problems with urine evacuation and may encourage urinary infections, kidney stone production, as well as major fatigue.

Most of the other organs are not displaced but will lose their normal mobility. This is why an x-ray (except for the kidneys) or MRI cannot show this type of pathology. Most of the medical examinations are static (immobile), and what we are looking at requires dynamic (mobile) examinations.

What about Emotions?

We have seen that emotions create visceral reactions. Suppose in your job you have a lot of frustrations that affect you directly. You can create a stomach irritation, and your brain will receive a combination of psychological and physical information. It will be very difficult to determine what is emotional and what is physical, and a vicious cycle will be created. With the Visceral Manipulation, the tension around the stomach will be released. Your brain will receive less negative information; therefore, you can break this vicious cycle. Of course, the opposite is also true. You can release the emotional component, and the organ will be less affected.

Does It Take Long to Get Results?

The time that it takes to see results will vary depending on the symptoms, the severity of symptoms, length of time that the symptoms have been bothering a person, etc. However, a person will usually start to feel results within three to five sessions.

Suppose you have hepatitis—your liver is sensitive, rigid, larger than normal, and has restricted movement. The therapist will feel a lack of mobility and a hardness when palpating the organ, so he knows he can do something physically. After three to five sessions he should feel that the liver is moving more and is softening. Above all, the patient should feel that his/her digestion is improving and that they are less fatigued.

When to See a Therapist

When you have symptoms like poor digestion, abdominal or pelvic pain, difficulty breathing, dorsal and low back pain, and sciatic pain, it is important to check with your physician to ensure that you do not have a serious illness which needs to be addressed. If they do not find a serious illness, it is important to see a Visceral Manipulation therapist, as our experience and research have shown that you can benefit from this treatment. It is also important to have a Visceral Manipulation check-up even if you don't have symptoms. Pathologies occur in the body long before we ever feel the symptoms. Prevention is the key.

How to Find a Visceral Manipulation Therapist

Thousands of therapists worldwide have now been trained to various degrees in Visceral Manipulation. Medical Doctors, Osteopathic Physicians, Chiropractors, Physical Therapists, Rolfers, Massage Therapists, Occupational Therapists, and many other types of bodyworkers are qualified to practice Visceral Manipulation. However, as with any therapy, it is important that you make sure the therapist is properly trained.

NOTE: Due to the international popularity of Jean-Pierre Barral's work over the past twenty years, the Barral Institute was formed. The Barral Institute offers qualified therapists recognized training programs in Visceral Manipulation taught by certified Visceral Manipulation Instructors.

For more information about Jean-Pierre Barral, The Barral Institute, and any of its programs, as well as to find a qualified Visceral Manipulation therapist in your area, you can contact The Barral Institute directly at www.barralinstitute.com.

ABOUT THE AUTHOR ‿⁊

D R. JEAN-PIERRE BARRAL was trained at the European School of Osteopathy in Maidstone, England. A well-known clinician and teacher in his native France and throughout Europe, he has authored many osteopathic textbooks. His works in English include *Visceral Manipulation* (with Pierre Mercier, DO), *Visceral Manipulation II, The Thorax, Urogenital Manipulation, Manual Thermal Evaluation,* and most recently *Trauma: An Osteopathic Approach.*

TIME magazine (UK) named Jean-Pierre Barral, DO, one of the top 100 practitioners in alternative medicine to watch for in the new millennium in the 1999 feature, "Innovators: TIME 100 The Next Wave, Alternative Medicine."

Dr. Barral is presently Academic Director of the International College of Osteopathy in Saint Etienne, France, and the Chairman of the Department of Visceral Manipulation on the Faculty of Medicine at Paris du Nord. He practices osteopathy in Grenoble, France.